Overcoming Obesity

Overcoming Obesity

Thomas V. Taylor, M.D., F.A.C.S., F.R.C.S., F.A.C.G.

Academic Chief of Surgery, St. Joseph Hospital, Houston

VANTAGE PRESS
New York

The opinions expressed herein are solely those of the author.
Each individual should seek the advice of his or
her own physician before beginning any new
health, diet, or medical program.

Cover design by Polly McQuillen

FIRST EDITION

Published by Vantage Press, Inc.
419 Park Ave. South, New York, NY 10016

Manufactured in the United States of America
ISBN: 978-0-533-15475-3

Library of Congress Catalog Card No.: 2006901853

0 9 8 7 6 5 4 3 2 1

Contents

List of Figures

Acknowledgments

I would like to express my sincere thanks to Sandra Hajtman for her encouragement, dedication, and help in the production of this book. Also to Dr. Margo Restrepo, Chief of Psychiatry at St. Joseph Medical Center in Houston, Texas, for contributing the sections on psychology and psychiatry.

I would also like to thank Dr. Stephen Holt, my longtime friend and colleague, for his help and encouragement. Thanks are also due to Kay McKeough and Dorothy Knox Houghton for their editorial support.

Overcoming Obesity

I

Obesity—The Size and Cost of the Problem

Definition

The word "obesity" refers to an excess of body fat. An excess of body fat is defined as a body mass index of 28 kg/m^2 or body weight 20 percent or more above ideal body weight (Table 1). Some thirty-four million adults in the United States are obese by this definition. Of these, six million have a body mass index of over 40 kg/m^2, meaning that they suffer from severe or morbid obesity, the risks of which are life threatening. This number has doubled in the last ten years and continues to increase rapidly.

Incidence

The rates of obesity are increasing among Americans of all ages, ethnicities and socioeconomic groups. Presently they are highest among African Americans and Hispanics. One of the most alarming statistics is that one in six American children between the ages of six and nineteen years is now obese. Between 1996 and 2001, two million teenagers and young adults joined the ranks of the clinically obese. Americans spend thirty two billion dollars per year on diets and weight reducing methods. The annual medical costs related to obesity are estimated at over sixty billion dollars. The value of time lost from work as a direct result of obesity amounts to an additional forty billion dollars per year. All of this has had very little impact on the underlying problem. The average person in the United States consumes some 150 lbs. of refined sugar per year and excess sugar consumption is directly related to obesity.

The United States is a very body conscious country. Its public face, as depicted on magazine covers, in movies and on television, is of youth, vitality and sexual attractiveness. In reality, however, fewer and fewer Americans resemble this hallmark.

History

In the industrial era, hard physical labor and periodic economic privation discouraged weight gain. Only the privileged leisure class had the opportunity to grow fat. Protective genetic traits that once defended the hearty from starvation now make those same persons susceptible to becoming overweight. At the same time, many people remain immersed in the socioeconomic issues of their families of origin, where unlimited access to food and plumpness were once commonly associated with success and prosperity. Today, the car and computer rule our lives, thrusting the majority into a "leisure class" that lacks physical activity and has relatively unlimited access to food. Too many people are so focused on surviving economically in a "fast forward" world that time for exercise has long since been lost.

Table 1

Body Mass Index $= \dfrac{\text{Weight in Kilograms}}{(\text{Height in meters})^2}$

Obesity	BMI > 25	Overweight
	BMI 30–40	Obese
Morbid Obesity	BMI > 40	
Super Obesity	BMI > 50	

II

The Nature of the Problem

Body Fat

Measuring the exact amount of fat in the body is difficult. X-ray and electrical methods are complex and tend to be inaccurate. The most commonly used measure of obesity is the Body Mass Index (BMI) defined as the ratio of the weight in kilograms to the square of the height, in meters. A BMI of 25 to 29.9 indicates that a patient is overweight. A person with a BMI of over 30 is considered obese and those over 40 are described as being "morbidly obese" (Table 1).

Syndrome X

Obesity is more than a cosmetic problem. It is the direct cause of a host of the medical problems which are the biggest killers of American citizens today. The three most important problems associated with the obese state are high blood pressure, high blood cholesterol, and diabetes mellitus. This trio is often referred to as Syndrome X (Table 2). Seventy million Americans suffer from Syndrome X, the components of which are all linked by sugar intolerance due to insulin resistance. This collection of problems now represents the number one public health initiative facing Western society. This disorder is much more common than AIDS and cancer and is the mechanism by which we, in Western society, have created a new constellation of killer diseases from which we all suffer to a variable degree.

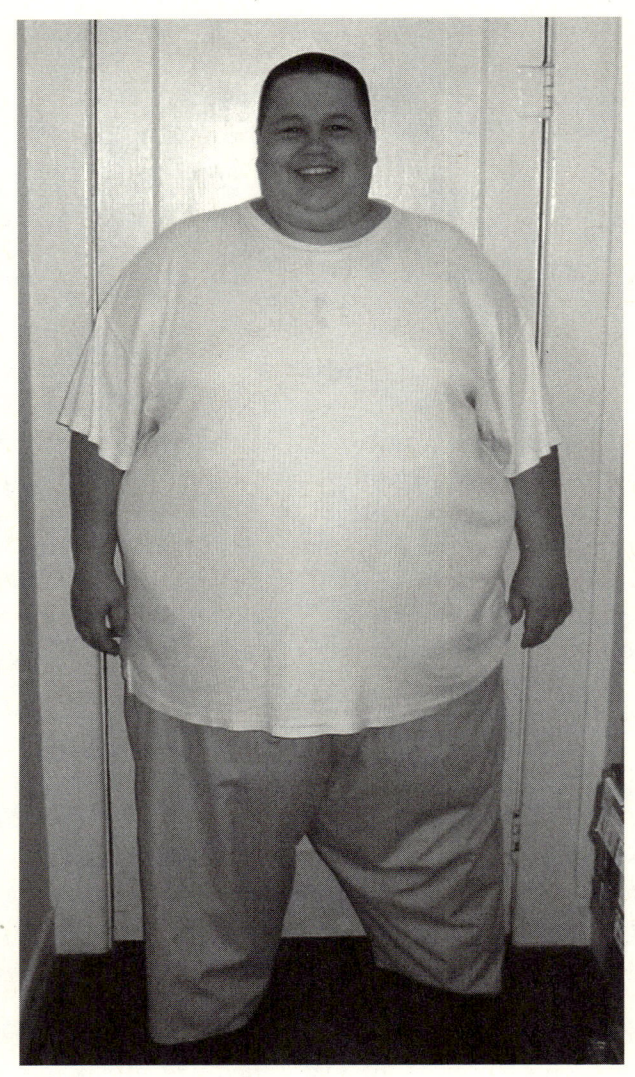

Figure 1

Tom, who struggles with morbid obesity

Table 2

Syndrome X

- High blood pressure (hypertension)
- High blood cholesterol
- Diabetes mellitus

Lifestyle

Our current lifestyle and behavior is largely responsible for this problem. The lifestyle is sedentary; watching television, sitting in front of computers and driving everywhere. Over the past century, technological developments have almost completely removed physical exercise from our day-to-day lives. In association with diet, this lifestyle sets the scene for the major killers: coronary artery disease, stroke, diabetes and several forms of cancer (Table 3). The syndrome now affects not only the elderly or the middle-aged, it is having a major affect on children and teenagers.

Table 3

Consequences of Syndrome X

1. Coronary artery disease
2. Stroke (cerebro-vascular accident)
3. Complications of diabetes mellitus
4. Some forms of cancer, breast, colon and ovary

Changes in the Past Century

Mankind has evolved over millions of years but only in the last century has change developed at an unrelenting pace never before experienced. We have walked the roads to and from our destinations day in, day out, for many millions of years. In the past few thousand years, the fastest mode of transportation had been the horse. In the past century we have developed the technology to travel the world in a day—New York to Australia. We have also become dependent upon mechanization in every walk of life. Buses to school, cars to work, engines to dig and till the soil, to build roads and buildings and manufacture goods. The effect of lying in front of a screen eating and drinking carbohydrate-laced foods has been to create a new model of human. Our supermarket shelves are packed with cheap, mass produced, good tasting, readily available food which is very high in calories. These foods are constantly attractively displayed in advertisements on the televisions, to which we have become glued.

Geography & Western Lifestyle

Interestingly, people who migrate to the U.S. from poorer areas such as Latin American and Asia adopt these Western lifestyles and become obese. Improved nutrition has done much to enhance human performance, physical and possibly intellectual performance, but modern nutrition has also created Syndrome X, which is killing us. Syndrome X is caused by a disturbance of body chemistry emanating from lack of exercise and the consumption of refined sugars. Think of a one pound bag of refined sugar, think of 150 bags in a pile; this is how much sugar the average person consumes per year. Cans of soda contain about 200 calories per drink, all of which are sugar—refined carbohydrate. There is the equivalent of nine teaspoons of sugar in a can of soda (Figure 2).

Sugar Is the Major Cause

Eating our way through this mountain of sugar is the primary cause of heart attacks, vascular disease, strokes and diabetes. Other health problems which ensue are breast and colon cancer and menstrual abnormalities (polycystic ovary syndrome which is also associated with female infertility), unwanted body hair and acne. Inflammation of the liver, increased tendency for blood to clot and depression of the immune system may also occur. These disorders are those of the twentieth century, those of modern living. Coronary artery disease, stroke and diabetes were all rare in the nineteenth century. Admittedly many people died at a younger age,

FIGURE 2 **Average Per Capita Sugar Consumption in the U.S.A.**

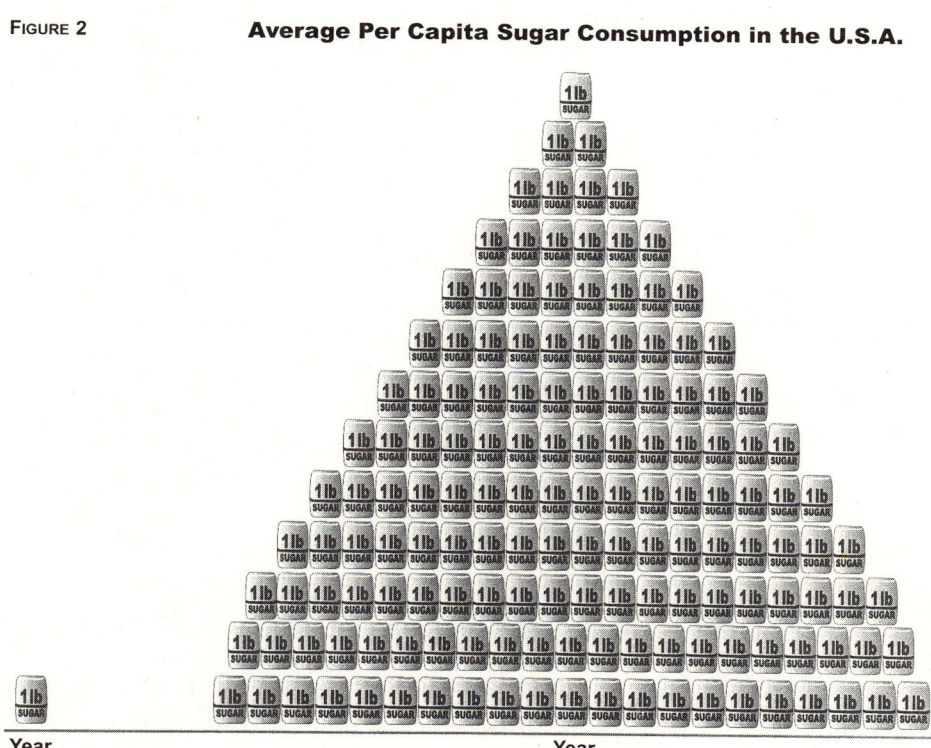

Year
1900

Year
2000

Annual sugar consumption in the U.S.A.

7

often of infectious diseases such as tuberculosis and pneumonia. In certain parts of the world these former diseases are rare today.

The Western Diet

The common gastrointestinal conditions which surgeons treat today are all self-induced by the high-sugar, low-fiber diet (Table 4). Gallstones, diverticular disease, appendicitis, hemorrhoids and colon cancer are extremely rare in Central Africa where a diet high in fiber and unrefined carbohydrates is prevalent. Take the Central African out of his own environment and put him into the United States, however, and he will soon develop the same disorders as the American population.

Table 4

Gastrointestinal Diseases Caused by Sugar

- Gallstones
- Diverticular disease
- Appendicitis
- Hemorrhoids
- Colon cancer

Taking Hunting from the Hunter-Gatherer Equation

Our earliest ancestors probably ate foods similar to those eaten by apes and monkeys. These were: fruits, shoots, nuts, tubers and other vegetation in the forests of Africa. Most of these plants were relatively low in calories and took constant work to collect them and thus stay alive. Early mankind began eating meat some 2.5 million years ago and the fossil record shows that the human brain became remarkably bigger and more complex at about the same time. The incorporation of animal matter into the diet played an essential role in human evolution. The fatty acids found in meat played an important role in brain growth.

Meat Is Good for the Brain

The high concentration of nutrients in meat gave humans some respite from constantly gathering and eating vegetation. In parallel the growth of the brain produced guile, cunning and organization which led to the development of technology and socialization. The meat our ancestors ate was high in protein and low in fat (4 percent). Also the supply was sporadic and a lot of energy was expended in catching it, leading to a lean body habitus.

III

The Basis of Obesity

Laws of Energy

Sir Isaac Newton, the father of modern physics, stated that energy cannot be created or destroyed but only converted from one form to another. Energy exists in many different forms—oil and food are forms of chemical energy. Burning oil permits planes to fly, cars to run, houses to be heated and cooled and electricity to be generated. Burning food permits us to live, to run, to walk, to talk and do our many lifetime activities. The energy which isn't actively being burned in a plane or a car is stored in the fuel tank. Oil is a form of fat. When the tanks are empty the vehicle stops.

Sources of Energy

Man derives energy from three sources: protein, carbohydrate and fat. We are extremely efficient in the collection, storage and utilization of energy, much more so than planes or cars. The energy taken in food is either utilized or stored. In the process of staying alive, maintaining our bodies and our body temperatures, we use energy of the order of 1,500 calories per day (Table 5). When we work, play sports and partake in other activities, we burn up the additional energy needed for these physical processes. We can utilize 2,000—3,000 calories per day (differences of caloric needs exist for men versus women) or even more than that. Physical exercise for example, riding a bicycle for an hour typically burns only 300 to 400 calories, but exercise is important in the energy equation.

Table 5

Basal Metabolic Rate (BMR)

This is minimal energy expenditure or energy usage while completely resting.

BMR	—Females	1,200–1,500 calories
	—Males	1,500– 2,000 calories

According to Newton's laws, any energy which our body doesn't burn, it stores. Protein provides four calories per gram, sugar likewise, whereas a gram of fat contains nine calories. The human body has fuel tanks like a plane or a car. These fuel tanks are made almost entirely of solid fat.

Energy Storage

The body does not act as a storage organ for protein. Weight-lifters and "muscle men" store some energy in their increased muscle mass but not a lot. Likewise the body is a poor storage organ for carbohydrate. There is some carbohydrate in muscle and about 150 grams in the liver, stored as a chemical, called glycogen. The body stores of glycogen are about 600 calories or the equivalent of about two hours of riding on a bike. Clearly after two hours on a bike the Lance Armstrongs of this world do not collapse in a state of energy depletion, they begin to use fat. The fat stores of the body are not only extremely efficient they have the potential to be huge.

If we eat more than we burn—Newton's laws again—we store the excess energy not as protein or carbohydrate but as fat. Unlike the fuel tanks on a vehicle, unfortunately, the fat stores in man do not become replete once they have enough energy for a long journey, they can just keep on growing.

Fat Is the Vehicle of Energy Storage

A morbidly obese subject does not have a frame size much bigger than that of a skinny person. He or she has the same amount

11

of bone, a little more muscle, the same sized brain, the same lungs and guts and a little bigger heart for all the extra work it has to do. If the basic frame of a 600 lb man is 150 lbs then he is carrying 450 pounds of fat, and carrying it twenty-four hours a day—every time he moves, every time he walks, every time he climbs stairs. That is the equivalent of carrying about four large sacks of grain on his back every time he moves. These "sacks of grain" strain the heart, the lungs, the muscles, the bones and the joints.

Excess calories are rapidly converted to fat because they cannot be lost if they are not burned. As fat contains nine calories per gram a steady excess caloric intake over our needs of 1000 calories per day, will lead to a weight gain of approximately 100 grams per day or about two pounds per week. Not much—well two pounds per week is 100 lbs in a year. An excess of 1000 calories per day is easily achieved and amounts to four cans of soda or four relatively small chocolate bars. And remember it takes over two hours of cycling to burn it off. Thus consistently eating just a little in excess of one's needs can have serious consequences.

Carbohydrate Produces Body Fat

In the process of food absorption and metabolism excess carbohydrate intake is ultimately converted into and stored as fat. Similarly, alcohol, which is energy dense, eight calories per gram, is also stored as fat, even protein excesses are stored as fat.

The Obesity Industry

In general therefore, it is true to say that "individuals who eat in excess of their needs will tend to be overweight and those who do not eat enough will tend to be underweight."

Sixty percent of Americans are overweight and a few are underweight. In consequence, weight control and obesity management are among the largest industries in North America and it is estimated that about one quarter of the population expends about $30 billion on weight control aids each year. Approximately 20 percent of the population describe themselves as being on some form of diet and three quarters of mid-teenage girls try to control their weight or lose weight. The vast majority of obese children become obese teenagers and most obese teenagers become obese adults and remain obese adults throughout their lives. Once the thermostat of weight creeps up to a high level it rarely stabilizes back to normal in the long term, unless some major intervention takes place permanently to affect the equation, and that currently means surgical intervention to reduce food intake and alter metabolism.

Sugar Is the Enemy

Historically much lip service was paid to the low-fat diet. The philosophy was often one of avoiding fat and giving "carte blanche" to the ingestion of carbohydrates. This has now been turned around, largely by the pioneering work of the late Robert Atkins, who popularized the low, or virtually "no" carbohydrate diet. When it was introduced, his philosophy flew in the face of established thinking and was soundly condemned in many academic circles but the proof of the pudding, in particular, was in the eating! The bottom line for millions has been that the Atkins diet results in weight loss and even a reduction in cholesterol and an amelioration of obesity and Syndrome X. Sugar is the enemy. Sugar is toxic.

Sugar & Insulin

Sugar is an easily absorbed and pleasant to eat source of rapid energy but it has bad effects by directly stimulating insulin production. Insulin causes our bodies to store excess sugar as fat and it inhibits the mobilization of previously stored fat. In addition, insulin signals our livers to make cholesterol. That's why even when eating the high cholesterol content foods of the Atkins diet, levels of blood cholesterol fall, as there is less insulin production. Diabetic patients have significantly higher total cholesterol and triglycerides than the normal population. It is for these reasons that modern diets like the Atkins diet, the South Beach diet and the Sugar Busters diets drastically reduce the amount of refined carbohydrate which can be eaten.

Counting Carbs

As recently stated in *Time Magazine*, "Counting carbs has become as powerful a fixture in the economy as it has in society."

Some 586 distinct new low-carb foods and beverages hit the grocery shelves in the last quarter of 2004, bringing the total over two years to 1,558 new entries. This is having a major effect on the food giants as "carb watching" would appear to be here for the long term. Things may be changing! It is possible that the effects of carb counting are beginning to become established in America. It was reported in the last year that after six consecutive years of weight gain the number of overweight adult Americans fell 1 percentage point, to 55 percent. In parallel, in fast food restaurants the total number of orders rose twelve percent, while French-fry consumption fell ten percent. National potato production has also fallen by five percent.

IV

The Consequences of Obesity

Diabetes in Children

The presence of obesity stimulates the development of type 2 diabetes previously regarded as the adult form. Even in children and adolescents this is increasingly being observed. In afflicted children and adolescents the type of diabetes is changing. It used to be that children got the more aggressive, often inherited, type 1 diabetes. Now in addition they are developing type 2 diabetes. In a ten-year period there has been a staggering 500 percent increase in type 2 diabetes and these children are invariably obese.

The prevalence of type 2 diabetes in Americans has escalated exponentially so that now more than twenty states have a prevalence of obesity of greater than 20 percent of the population.

Cost of Obesity

The Surgeon General's report estimated the costs of obesity to be $117 billion in the year 2001. One half of this money is spent on treating the complications of diabetes, or other conditions produced by diabetes, such as heart attacks, stroke, kidney failure and blindness (Table 6). We hear so much of the detrimental effects of smoking and drinking but diabetes outranks both of these in its deteriorating effects on health.

Table 6

Complications of Diabetes

- Heart attacks, myocardial infarction
- Stroke, cerebrovascular accidents
- Renal (kidney) failure
- Retinopathy (visual failure)
- Neuropathy (nerve damage)

Type 2 Diabetes

Type 2 diabetes can be prevented or reversed by weight reduction and lifestyle modification. Remarkably it is cured immediately in the vast majority who undergo obesity surgery. Obesity surgery also cures Syndrome X and other problems associated with Syndrome X, namely high cholesterol and blood pressure.

The Sugar-Insulin Relationship

Insulin production and utilization is the key to diabetes, which allows sugars to enter the cell and provide energy. When the lock is faulty, sugars cannot enter the cells and they build up in the bloodstream, where they cause damage. Carrying excess fat adds to the difficulty which insulin has in doing its job. If the sugar cannot enter the cells the pancreas goes on pumping out more and more insulin in response to the high blood sugar. Ultimately the insulin may overshoot the mark and produce a rapid fall in blood sugar which causes powerful appetite stimulation (Table 7).

Table 7

Insulin

- A hormone secreted by the pancreas
- Permits sugar to enter the cell
- Controls energy
- Too little causes diabetes and high blood sugar
- Too much can cause behavioral changes leading to coma
- Stimulates appetite
- Converts carbohydrates into fat particles

Diabetics whose blood sugar is poorly controlled are continuously pouring out excess insulin to which they become increasingly resistant. The high levels of blood sugar damage other organs, in particular the eye and the kidney, leading to blindness and renal failure. Extremes of blood sugar concentrations, both low and high, may lead to coma which is life threatening. Diabetics also develop accelerated arteriosclerosis with a risk of heart attacks, strokes and gangrene.

Glucagon

A second important hormone, glucagon, which is secreted in the pancreas, acts in many ways as an opposite to insulin. Glucagon is released by a protein stimulus, not glucose. Glucagon promotes the mobilization of previously stored fat, so you burn body fat in response to this hormone rather than store it in response to insulin. Carbohydrate-rich meals suppress glucagon secretion.

The continued excessive stimulus to insulin production created by the high carbohydrate diet ultimately produces insulin resistance, which is a diminished effect of insulin in response to more sugar.

Refined Carbohydrates

Ancient man, for many thousands of years, ate unrefined carbohydrates as part of the hunter-gatherer type of diet. With these diets, the pancreas was stimulated to a much lesser extent than with current diets. Until 200 years ago humans ate less than one pound of refined sugar per year, now, as stated, 150 pounds are eaten per year. Sugar manufacturers, cola producers and the packaged food industry have paved the way to the current situation. However cynical it may sound, the sugar manufacturers have contributed to the deaths of more Americans than all wars combined.

Glucose

We eat carbohydrates in the form of simple sugars and starches. All carbohydrates are eventually broken down to the simple sugar glucose. Glucose maintains the blood sugar at a steady level in the non-diabetic. Small amounts (600 grams) are stored in the liver, and to a lesser extent, in muscle. Any remaining glucose is converted to and stored as fat.

Starches

Complex starches are absorbed less rapidly, and are slowly broken down to glucose. It is the rapid absorption of ingested refined carbohydrates which increase the blood sugar concentration and stimulate insulin secretion (Table 8).

Table 8

Blood Sugar

- Remains stable in normal individuals
- Increases in the diabetic
- Stimulates the release of insulin
- Glucagon counteracts the effect of insulin
- EXCESS SUGAR CONSUMPTION PRODUCES INSULIN RESISTANCE

Normal people secrete about 25 to 30 units of insulin per day. Insulin sweeps glucose into cells where it is stored. Insulin prevents the level of glucose in the blood from rising. Conversely, glucagon in the fasting state prevents the blood sugar from falling too low. Too much insulin can produce dangerously low levels of blood sugar.

Insulin Resistance

Excessive glucose intake over time produces insulin resistance. Then there is a decreased responsiveness to insulin wherein fat cells, liver cells and muscle cells become insensitive to insulin and blood glucose concentrations rise. Insulin resistance is a major factor in the development of obesity. The high levels of circulating insulin cause the body continually to store as much fat as is possible. Insulin resistance is also the fundamental problem underlying Syndrome X. Reducing the intake of sugar will lower the peak insulin levels and will ultimately reduce insulin resistance.

The precise reasons why insulin resistance occurs are not known. Insulin resistance can run in families and is made worse by unhealthy lifestyle habits. These habits are lack of exercise, poor diet with both nutritional deficiencies and excesses and substance abuse (smoking and drinking).

Fat, Cholesterol & Arteriosclerosis

One of the roles of insulin is to convert carbohydrates into minute fat particles called triglycerides. This predisposes to fat storage, to obesity and to heart disease. Triglyceride and cholesterol concentrations in the blood are the main predictive factors for arteriosclerosis. Basically there are two types of cholesterol, high and low density lipoprotein cholesterol. In the simplest of terms, high density lipoprotein cholesterol is good cholesterol and low density lipoprotein cholesterol is bad cholesterol. The process of arteriosclerosis, or hardening of the arteries, begins with the development of streaks or plaques of cholesterol on the lining of blood vessels (Table 9). Subsequently these plaques become raised and hard, ultimately leading to a thrombosis or blockage of the artery. If this occurs in the coronary arteries it produces angina, a tight pain in the chest, sometimes radiating to the neck and arms,

19

which is often produced by exercise. The pain results from a lack of blood supply to the muscle of the heart. Ultimately the coronary arteries may become completely occluded. This is a condition known as coronary thrombosis which cuts off the blood supply to the heart muscle, and leads to death of the heart muscle or myocardial infarction. The most predictive factor for arteriosclerosis is hyperinsulinism.

Table 9

Arteriosclerosis

- Streaks or plaques of cholesterol are deposited on the lining of arteries
- Plaques become raised and hard
- Clots can develop on the plaque
- This produces thrombosis or blockage of the vessel
- Vessel blockage causes infarction or gangrene of tissues

Hypertension

Another problem associated with hyperinsulinism and high blood glucose levels is hypertension, or high blood pressure, also part of Syndrome-X. Most cases of hypertension are attributed to hyperinsulinism and this usually precedes the overtly diabetic state. Hypertension in itself predisposes to coronary artery disease, stroke and kidney failure.

Good Fats and Bad Fats

For many years the message about the ill effects of ingested fat prevailed. Fifty years ago the main villain, in terms of producing the rapidly increasing wave of heart attacks and strokes, was thought to be animal fat. There is however an increasing amount of evidence that unsaturated non-trans fats are good for us. These are not necessarily the fats in margarine, they are fats like olive oil.

The Omega Fatty Acids

It has long been known that Mediterranean races have a much lower incidence of coronary artery disease and stroke than northern Europeans. This may be related to a diet rich in unsaturated fats which contain omega-3 fatty acids. A commonly quoted study, the Lyons Heart Study, looked at a butter substitute, canola oil, which is mostly a monounsaturated fat with omega-3 fatty acids. In a series of patients, all of whom had previously had a heart attack, there was a 70 percent decrease in subsequent heart attacks in those who received the good fat. Another study, the GISSI Prevention Trial, showed that fish oil capsules—omega-3 fatty acids—decreased sudden deaths. Omega-3 fatty acids, plentiful in fish, seem to confer some protection against the development of heart attacks and strokes.

Capsules of omega-3 fatty acids in large doses are also effective in treating depressive illnesses. Additionally, a number of studies have shown that nuts, which contain a lot of unsaturated fats, are protective against heart attacks and strokes. Good fats are called essential fatty acids which fall into two main categories, the omega-3 and omega-6 groups. Omega-3 fatty acids are found in leaves and plant seeds, in egg yolks and in salmon, herring, tuna, cod and mackerel. Omega-6 fatty acids are found in plant seeds, especially black currants. There also are omega-9 fatty acids, the most plentiful of which, oleic acid, is found in olive oil, some nuts and avocados.

The American Heart Association has for many years stated that eating saturated fats such as butter and lard will accelerate the process of arteriosclerosis and lead to the clogging of arteries. Conversely, eating foods high in polyunsaturated fats was thought to keep the arteries clear. On the other hand, Robert Atkins came out in strong defiance of the dictum. Even the famous long-standing, and most often quoted study, the Framingham Study, realized there was uncertainty surrounding this stance.

Supporting Atkins's position, Ceștelli has stated, "We found that the people who ate the most cholesterol, or the most saturated fat, or the most calories from fat, weighed the least and were physically the most active."

The combined evidence to date raises serious questions about the role of dietary saturated fats in causing heart disease and the supposed role of polyunsaturated fatty acids in preventing it.

Balancing the Fats

Healthy fat intake almost certainly depends upon getting the correct proportions of the various fats in the diet. The modern American diet has led to a serious imbalance in the ratio of omega-3 to omega-6 fatty acids. This is a result of consuming a lot of refined corn, soy, sunflower and canola oils, which contain large amounts of omega-6 fatty acids and relatively small amounts of omega-3 fatty acid. In contrast, for centuries the source of essential fatty acids was omega-3 rich whole grains, nuts, vegetables and egg yolks.

Diet, Race and Heart Disease

Native Greenlanders have lived traditionally on a diet that consists of meat and blubber from seals and whales. These mammals feed on fish whose flesh has a high concentration of omega-3 fatty acids. Omega-3 fatty acids lower triglycerides and LDL cholesterol. Furthermore, they lower blood pressure and have an anticoagulant effect, thus preventing coronary artery thrombosis and stroke. Heart disease is extremely rare in the classical indigenous Greenland native. Several studies have shown that eating fish reduces deaths from heart disease.

Alcohol

Alcohol, at eight calories per gram, is rich in energy. Most diets ban alcohol but alcohol appears to be good for longevity in wine producing and consuming countries. A glass of wine has fewer calories than a slice of white bread (Table 10). Beer is widely seen as bad news for anyone counting calories, maltose adds to carbohydrate calories. Beer sales have declined slightly while sales of spirits increased by three percent last year. Calories absorbed from alcohol are readily available for utilization as energy and therefore may block fat consumption. Alcohol may also act as an appetite stimulant. In terms of calorie intake, the liquor is not always the problem, it is the soda mixer that goes with it. Stores are now beginning to sell products like "Baja Bob's low-carb margarita mix" and bars are stocking more diet sodas. Low carb beers are also proliferating. Ultra was introduced in 2002 and sales have more than quadrupled.

Table 10

Alcohol

- Eight calories per gram (fat is 9 calories per gram)
- Red wine, up to two glasses per day is healthy
- Red wine protects against vascular disease
- Beer is contraindicated, it has a high glycemic index—maltose
- A bottle of spirits contains two days' supply of calories

V

Long-term Hazards of Obesity

It has been known since the 1950s that men between the ages of thirty and thirty-nine had a progressive increase in mortality with increasing weight. The increase began with weights just in excess of the acceptable weight range. Overall mortality in obese men increases with age thereafter.

Reduced Life Expectancy

Excess weight gain in females is also associated with increased mortality, which begins at a somewhat older age than in men. Those overweight men and women who lose substantial amounts of weight and remain at a weight within the optimal range for an appreciable time appear to have a lower mortality risk than an equivalent group of overweight individuals. This adds further evidence to the conclusion that obesity decreases life span. The other measurable factor which has a major influence on longevity is smoking. In non-smoking men and women the risk of being 35 to 50 percent overweight respectively confers the same risk as smoking with a body weight within the acceptable range (Table 11).

Table 11

Risks of Obesity

Heart Attack
Hypertension
Stroke
High Cholesterol Levels
Diabetes Mellitus
Gallstones
Gout
Osteoarthritis
Kidney Stones
Cancer—Breast, Uterus, Cervix

Syndrome X

Obesity has been shown to have a significant role to play in the genesis of coronary artery disease. There are, however, other strong risk factors including age, male sex, hypertension, smoking and elevated cholesterol concentrations.

Some of these other risk factors, particularly high blood pressure and serum cholesterol, are directly related to obesity. Another factor related to heart disease and to obesity is physical inactivity, which has been scientifically shown in many studies to be related to the development of heart disease. It ultimately plays a role in obesity at all ages. It has been shown that both vigorous exercise and walking are protective not only from the point of view of containing developing obesity, but also, coronary artery disease. The exact mechanism of the protective effect is not fully understood. Studies on the role of blood pressure and the relationship between blood pressure and obesity are somewhat conflicting but there is good evidence that as weight increases with increasing age there is an elevation in blood pressure. In addition, evidence exists that weight loss results in a reduction in blood pressure. The relationship between obesity and diabetes is beyond question and diabetes is also a factor in the development of heart disease and hypertension (Table 12).

Table 12

Long-term Hazards of Obesity

Shortened Life Expectation
Diabetes Mellitus
Coronary Artery Disease
Heart Failure
Respiratory Failure
Liver Failure
Stroke
Osteoarthritis of Hips and Knees
Gallstones
Sleep Apnea
Kidney Stones
Gout
Deep Vein Thrombosis
Pulmonary Embolism
Dermatological Problems
Cellulitis
Infections and Septicemia
Cancer of Colon, Rectum, Prostate, Breast, Uterus and Cervix

Stone Formation

Kidney and gallstone formation are also closely related to obesity. Gallstones probably result from the ingestion of excessive amounts of cholesterol and changes in liver function which deposit more cholesterol in bile in the obese subject. Another factor which predisposes toward gallstone formation in the obese is the use of inappropriate slimming diets. Rapid reductions in weight or prolonged periods of starvation undoubtedly predispose toward the development of gallstones.

Joint Disease

Gout is a complication of obesity, the incidence of which increases in those over 130 percent of their appropriate weight. Sufferers from gout develop uric acid stones in their kidneys. Osteoarthritis is a very common condition which occurs increasingly with increasing weight. This is a wear and tear process of the cartilage which lines joints, producing erosion and damage to the joint space with exposure of bone to bone within the joint space. Usually it occurs as a result of damage to the joints which are most vulnerable to the obese state, in particular the hips and knee joints. Arthritis produces joint pain and restricts exercise tolerance thus creating a vicious circle leading to further weight gain.

Cancer

The American Cancer Society has shown an association between obesity and increased risk of cancer of the colon, rectum and prostate. With increasing weight, women show a progressive increase in the risk of cancer of the breast, uterus and cervix.

Heart and Lung Disease

Obesity places considerable burden on the heart and respiratory system. Lung function becomes increasingly impaired with increasing weight. It further impairs exercise tolerance and ultimately the morbidly obese patient with a combination of heart, lung and joint disease becomes beleaguered and totally unable to perform any form of exercise. Even walking or climbing stairs becomes severely restricted.

Another very common problem in association with obesity is sleep apnea. Sleep apnea is a condition in which levels of oxygen within the bloodstream fall, leading to sleep fragmentation, frequent wakening, and ultimately to the development of right-sided heart failure. This is associated with maladies of brain function which may occur as a result of damage to the central nervous system. The course of this condition is chronic and progressive. It is entirely reversible by weight loss.

Tobacco

People who smoke cigarettes are significantly lighter than non-smokers. Differences are often greatest in the lower income groups. It is well documented that body weight increases when smokers give up their habit and this unfortunately is often used by smokers as a reason to persist. While smoking is an appetite suppressant, the explanation for the weight gain that occurs when smoking is stopped may be related either to an increase in energy intake or a fall in energy expenditure. Smokers who give up the habit are particularly prone to take sweets and snacks. These are considered to form a substitute for a cigarette. It is also considered that cigarette smoking increases the metabolic rate, possibly by stimulating the sympathetic nervous system with nicotine.

VI

The Future—A Potential Decline in Life Expectancy as a Result of Obesity

Forecasts of life expectancy form an important component of government strategy with regard to such programs as Social Security and Medicare. Until recently, all forecasts of life expectancy favored a continuing increase. For the past 1,000 years there has been a slow and steady increase in life expectancy, occasionally punctuated by epidemics, famines and major wars. The risk of major pandemics has declined after the influenza outbreak at the end of World War I, which killed more people than the war. Gains in life expectancy at older ages are now much smaller than they were in the first half of the twentieth century. Some prognostications of life expectancy have been overly optimistic. The United Nations forecasted a projected life expectancy of 100 years for males and females in developed countries by the year 2300. The Social Security Administration arrived at a figure of life expectancy reaching the mid eighties later this century.

The Life-shortening Effect of Obesity

The above forecasts are now seriously being questioned as a result of the unprecedented increase in obesity in the United States. If current trends continue they will undoubtedly threaten to diminish the health and life expectancy of current and future generations. As has been stated, two-thirds of adults in the United States today are obese or overweight and fifty percent of African Americans are currently obese. As stated in an article in the *New England Journal of Medicine* in April, 2005, children and ethnic minorities have shown the greatest increase in obesity. These trends have affected all major racial and ethnic groups and all socioeconomic strata. It is now estimated that obesity causes approximately a quarter of a million deaths per year in the United States. The risk of developing diabetes in the United States has risen exponentially to between 30 and 40 percent. The life-shortening effect of diabetes is approximately thirteen years. If the prevalence of obesity continues to rise it will lead to an elevated risk of associated morbidities with a negative effect on longevity. Obesity reduces life expectation by between five and twenty years and increases with increasing excess weight. A continued rise in the prevalence of obesity could for the first time in 1,000 years lead to a statistical downturn in longevity for the whole population.

Other Threats to Increased Longevity

There are other realistic threats to increases in life expectancy, such as an increase in the AIDS epidemic, the development of infectious diseases which are resistant to antibiotics and the emergence of aggressive new strains of virus such as the influenza virus, the latest variant of which is referred to as the "bird flu." Infectious diseases have, over the centuries, always presented the greatest threat to life expectation. Another major threat has been famine, but now for the first time the major and probably inevitable threat to increased longevity relates directly to the presence of obesity in today's society.

VII
The Basic Causes of Obesity

Why do people become excessively obese? The essential answer is because, in the long term, they ingest calories significantly in excess of their needs. It has been shown that the obese inherit a lower metabolic rate than normal weight individuals but as they gain weight the metabolic rate goes up to compensate and provide energy for the maintenance of their excess weight (Table 13).

Table 13

Q. Why Do People Become Obese?
A. Because they consistently take in more calories than they burn. There is no other easy answer!
Q. Why Is Obesity Becoming So Common?
  - Because of lifestyle changes
  - Eating the wrong food
  - Sitting in front of computers and televisions
  - Being influenced by food advertisements
  - Taking no exercise

Obesity Is Not Genetic—It's Behavioral

Obesity often begins early in life; there has been a doubling in the incidence of obesity in three- and four-year-olds in the last decade. During this time there has been no change in birth weight and no change in the gene pool, thus obesity in children is acquired and relates primarily to lifestyle. Factors which contribute to this are: The increased consumption of fast foods and high calorie carbohydrate drinks; reduced physical activity brought on by television viewing; food advertising and less breast feeding. These factors are strongly influenced by parents.

31

The Power of Advertising

Advertising is a powerful factor in this vicious equation. Food marketers target children and adults to influence their food choices and eating behavior. So lucrative is this business that one large company contracts to provide free computers and televisions to schools in exchange for compelling the children to view two minutes of commercial messages each day. Food advertising makes up a large proportion of this viewing time. This, perhaps, reflects on the way in which the nation's schools are funded. In relative terms education has become increasingly poorly financed. Furthermore the effects of the advertising campaigns are surreptitious and difficult to evaluate. We are all immersed in a sea of advertising, to a much greater degree than we are aware. If advertising was not so influential, companies would not invest in it, but observation of the plethora of advertising on television, the Internet, in the press and on our streets only goes to emphasize its relevance.

Schools—Starting on the Wrong Track

In the past decade, in some school districts, fast food companies took over school food service operations. Under these circumstances the fast-food company eliminates the burden to the school of providing meals that the child will eat. The question of appropriate nutrition, physical activity and weight management never entered the equation. These meal services are often supplemented by vending machines which provide an endless supply of sugar which is accessible throughout the day.

Between 1985 and 1997, soda sales to school distributors increased by 1,100 percent. Each can of soda contains the equivalent of ten teaspoons of sugar. One large soda drink can supply one-half of the total daily caloric count required by a teenager. The average child consumes in excess of one can of soda per day. A correlation exists between soda consumption and obesity in childhood. Soda consumption combined with an increasing lack of exercise is a potent combination in the production of obesity.

The above social factors driving obesity in childhood have been generated by and are equally present in the adult. Adults walk less, drive more cars, use more public transportation than ever before. There are more elevators, escalators, conveyer belts, televisions, computers and more couches. Conversely there are more gymnasiums, sales of exercise equipment, jogging tracks and other sports facilities. These latter, however are only used by a small pre-selected cross-section of the community but because of the physical encumbrance, produced by their excess fat, morbidly obese patients cannot use these aids.

Excess Energy Intake

The exact mechanism by which man controls his energy intake in order to maintain a steady weight is unknown. A "set point" seems to exist, which, in practical terms is a buffer zone around which most people keep their weight fairly constant (Table 14).

Table 14

The Set Point

- A point of stability around which the body weight remains stable
- Consistently eating more calories than are burned raises the set point
- Once elevated it is very difficult to get down again
- Is a buffer zone

The Set Point

Factors affecting this set point are: Satiety—a feeling of adequate food intake; neurohumoral factors; distension of the stomach; and the effects of stimulating the nerve fibers between the stomach and the brain. In trying to maintain the set point, the body intrinsically tries to control its calorie intake; increased intake, up to a point, stimulates activity whereas decreased intake tends to reduce physical activity through an expression of tiredness or induction of a restful state. It is possible for the body to reset the set point in an upward direction so that prolonged and continuous excess food intake produces elevation of the point of equilibrium. Conversely, defense of the set point has been used to explain why the maintenance of medically induced weight loss has been so poor.

Energy Conservation—Mode

Energy conservation is a factor which influences short-term weight stability. So often one hears from patients that they have virtually starved for a few days and not lost any weight. When fasting (conservation mode) the body probably reduces energy output by reducing metabolic rate to compensate for the sudden close off of food intake. This is probably not only confined to metabolic rate but also to energy usage by the body for exercise and day-to-day activities. Such conservation is probably related to the set point (Table 15).

Table 15

Energy Expenditure

Basal Metabolic Rate	1200 calories
Walking	250 cal/hour
Cycling	350 cal/hour
Running	400–600 cal/hour
Heavy Labor	400 cal/hour

(1 can of Coke—220 calories)

The Autonomic Nervous System

Energy expenditure is influenced to a large extent by activity generated by the sympathetic nervous system. The sympathetic nervous system may be likened to an electrical system of wiring which reaches the whole body. Its function is often illustrated by stating that it is the system by which our body responds by "fright, fight and flight." In other words, it is a system of physical activation. The chemicals which act as transmitters in the sympathetic

34

nervous system are adrenaline and related compounds. The functional counterpart to the sympathetic nervous system is called the parasympathetic system; its electrical pathways mainly run through the vagus nerve, a nerve which runs from the hypothalamus of the brain to the heart, lungs and intestines.

The hypothalamus, part of the base of the brain, is intimately related to appetite. Destruction of one area in the hypothalamus increases vagus nerve firing (parasympathetic) and decreases sympathetic activity. Stimulation of the vagus nerve triggers pancreatic insulin release and makes the stomach empty at a faster rate thus promoting obesity. Congenital abnormalities of the hypothalamus, such as the Prader-Willi syndrome, are associated with a morbidly obese state. In addition to factors that stimulate the parasympathetic nervous system, anything that inhibits sympathetic activity leads to weight gain. Different areas in the hypothalamus have differing effects on appetite; there is an area at the front and on the outside of the hypothalamus which when damaged causes a reduction in food intake and an increase in energy expenditure. Neurosurgeons have attempted to treat obesity by damaging this critical area in the brain. Studies of autonomic nervous system function have found that obese patients have a depression of both sympathetic and parasympathetic activity.

Hormonal Factors: Thyroid Hormone

Many who suffer from obesity feel that their underlying problem is hormonal or "glandular" and that the thyroid gland, in particular, is the source of the problem. There is no evidence that obese patients have a different thyroidal hormonal response to changes in energy than normal non-obese individuals. Underactivity of the thyroid gland, a condition called myxedema, will predispose to obesity just as the overactive state of thyrotoxicosis is associated with weight loss and increased sympathetic activity. It is for this reason that many have attempted to use thyroid hormone for the treatment of obesity. Increased levels of thyroid hormone increase the patient's metabolic rate and may also produce undesirable and potentially dangerous complications such as cardiac rhythmic disturbances which may lead to cardiac failure or even sudden death. Anxiety, tremor, sweating and palpitations are other side effects of the use of thyroid hormone. Where thyroxine has been used in the treatment of obesity the results have been unimpressive.

Corticosteroids

Cushing's Syndrome, which is due to excessive production of corticosteroids by the adrenal gland, may produce obesity but the condition is distinctly uncommon and rarely contributes to the problem in the obese patient (Table 16). Adrenalectomy in animals has been associated with weight loss.

Table 16

Cushing's Syndrome

Truncal Obesity.
Buffalo Hump.
Peripheral Purple Striae.
Muscle Wasting—Thin Limbs.
Hypertension.
Peptic Ulceration.

Sex Hormones

Sex hormones influence the accumulation and distribution of fat. Females, on the whole, have a higher percentage of body fat than males and most morbidly obese people are female. The distribution of fat is also different between the sexes. Males deposit fat on their central abdomens and become "pot bellied"; females concentrate the fat on their lower abdomen, buttocks and thighs, becoming "pear shaped" (Figure 3).

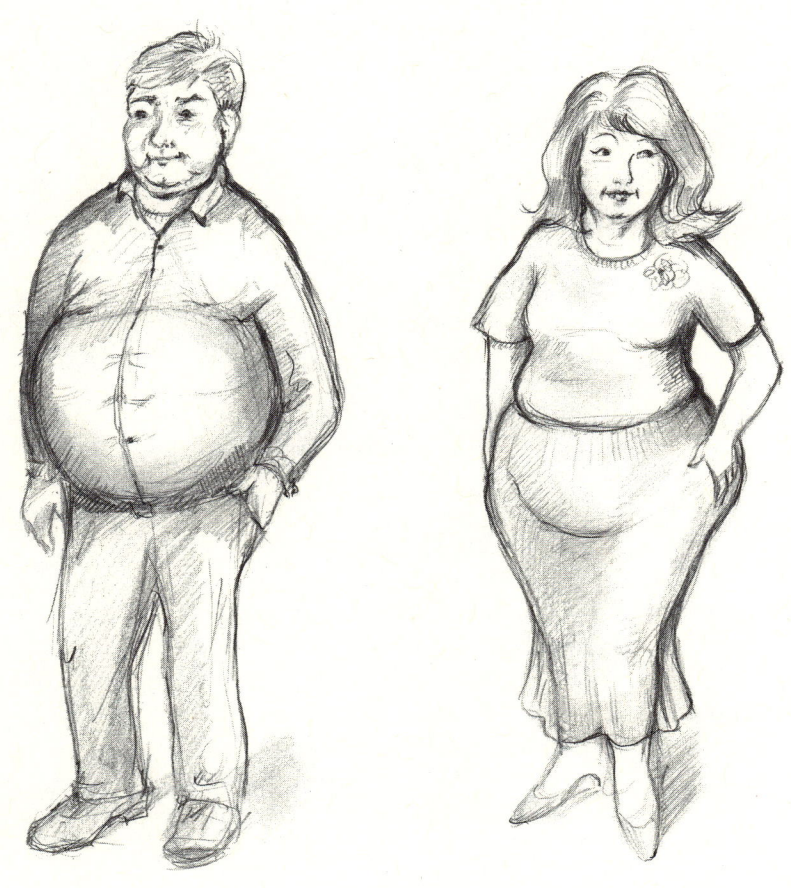

Figure 3

Distribution of fat in the male (apple) and female (pear)

Growth Hormone

Growth hormone has been advocated for use in weight loss programs and is also used in an attempt to preserve male strength and to prevent aging. The use of growth hormone does alter body habitus by redistributing fat and promoting muscle growth (Table 17).

Table 17

Excess Growth Hormone—Produces:

- Acromegaly
- Large size—gigantism
- Strong Muscles
- Large Hands
- Large Jaw
- Pituitary tumor can produce this

Gut Hormones

The gut produces many hormones often with variable action and interdependence, most of these decrease food intake. These hormones affect the secretion of acid and pancreatic juice; some have an influence on motility or contraction of the intestines. There is no real evidence that any of the hormones, under normal circumstances, play a significant role in the problem of obesity.

Below are listed naturally occurring chemicals which may affect the obese state (Table 18).

Table 18

Chemicals Related to the Obese State

- Leptin
- Resistin
- Neuropeptide-Y
- C-75
- Ghrelin

There have been several recent important observations which may assist in our understanding of the cause and treatment of obesity.

Ghrelin

In contrast to the other gut hormones a newly discovered substance, "ghrelin," increases food intake. Ghrelin, which is produced by the stomach, stimulates growth hormone release and causes excessive eating and obesity in rats. Levels of this hormone are, on the whole, lower in obese subjects but they do not decrease after a meal, as they do in subjects of normal weight.

Interestingly, levels of ghrelin in the body increase after dieting but are decreased by obesity surgery and this may therefore be a factor influencing weight loss after surgery. Ghrelin sends a signal to the brain to eat whenever the stomach is empty and to ease up when it is full. Some patients are now being experimentally treated with electronic pacemakers that apparently have a ghrelin-like effect convincing the stomach that it is fuller than it actually is.

C-75

The substance C-75 when administered to mice reduces food intake by ninety percent, C-75 treated mice lost 45 percent more weight than totally fasting animals. This is because C-75 inhibits feeding but does not decrease the metabolic rate or energy expenditure, as does fasting.

Neuropeptide-Y

Neuropeptide-Y is a naturally occurring substance in the brain which, when directly introduced into the brains of animals, produces voracious feeding. It is the most powerful appetite stimulant known. The substance inhibits thermogenesis, the heat generated by burning calories. During starvation neuropeptide-Y levels increase. Levels of insulin fall during starvation, and may help to stimulate a rise in neuropeptide-Y.

The action of neuropeptide-Y, which is completely blocked by C-75, is independent of leptin (vide infra). Neuropeptide-Y suppresses the sympathetic nervous system and produces marked weight gain in animals. The effects of this substance are mediated through a specific receptor in the brain, the so-called Y-receptor.

There have been several recent important observations which may assist in our understanding of the cause and treatment of weight loss.

Leptin

Leptin is one of half a dozen or so chemical messengers produced by fat cells, including clotting agents, blood vessel constricting agents and inflammatory agents that have powerful effects throughout the body.

Leptin is a protein gene which is defective in obese mice and obese humans. There is some evidence to suggest that replacement of leptin reverses obesity in animals. Studies in humans have been disappointing in their outcome. Leptin is thought to signal adequacy of food intake but high levels do little to turn off the stimulus to eat. When leptin was injected into mice, they suddenly changed their eating habits and began shedding fat. All mice have the leptin gene, but unfortunately it exists in only a handful of people. In those with the gene it has been shown to produce dramatic weight loss. In those that do not have the gene, it is pretty well ineffective. Some of the compounds discussed above like C-75 and neuropeptide-Y would, on theoretical grounds, at the present time, seem to offer more promise of a future therapeutic role than leptin. C-75 is a synthetic derivative of a naturally occurring substance called cerulenin. (Table 19)

Table 19

Ghrelin (from stomach)	tells the brain it is time to eat.
Cholecystokinin (from duodenum)	tells the brain it's time to stop.
Leptin & Insulin	Stabilizing factors—help to maintain the set point.

Resistin

A new hormone, "resistin," was discovered in 2001. This is a resistance to insulin hormone and is a protein molecule found in fat cells. The hormone is elevated in obesity and in insulin resistant patients. When fat cells are replete they release resistin, and insulin resistance ensues. However, the hormone is decreased in rodent obesity models and paradoxically increased by insulin-sensitizing drugs. A group of drugs, the thiazolidinediones, suppress the expression of resistin.

Orexins & Melanin-Stimulating Hormone

Orexins are substances found in the hypothalamus, which increase food intake. In contrast the substance melanocyte stimulating hormone from the pituitary gland inhibits food intake and results in weight loss.

Fat Storage

Fat storage evolved over millions of years as the primary mechanism for coping with periods of famine. For most of the period of evolution, the major problem was getting enough to eat in order to survive, rather than avoiding obesity. When calorie intake exceeds expenditure, fat cells swell to as much as six times their minimum size, and they begin to multiply. In the average adult there is something on the order of 40 billion fat cells which can increase up to 100 billion. Losing weight causes the fat cells to shrink in size and become less metabolically active, but their number goes down only very slowly, if at all.

Fat Cells, Inflammation and Immunity

The process of inflammation is currently receiving a lot of attention. Fat cells promote inflammation, which can spread throughout the body. Even small amounts of excess fat can produce a mounting immune response. This is because the body regards the storage of excess fat cells as an invading organism and attempts to reject it by mounting an inflammatory response. Inflammation is now viewed as a key mechanism in heart disease, probably being more important than cholesterol per se. Blood vessels such as the coronary arteries are undoubtedly narrowed by cholesterol but a big problem appears to be that an inflamed plaque can break open, produce clot and occlude a vessel—a process known as thrombosis.

In the case of the coronary arteries, this leads to the death of the heart muscle. Compounds secreted by fat cells contribute to vascular inflammation and they inhibit nitric oxide, a compound that helps relax blood vessel walls and lowers blood pressure. Fat cells also secrete estrogen, which is linked to certain types of cancer. Researchers now suspect that the origin of diabetes lies, at least partly, in the biochemistry of fat, in particular in two compounds made by fat cells. These are resistin and tumor necrosis factor alpha. Resistin promotes the conversion of fatty acids into glucose by the liver, a process that is useful during starvation, but a potential hazard in the obese patient. The amount of resistin which the body produces increases with the amount of fat stored. Tumor necrosis factor, a naturally occurring substance, promotes insulin resistance.

Fat cells behave differently in different parts of the body. Fat carried in the hips and thighs is considered comparatively benign whereas that which accumulates around organs in the abdomen is more harmful. The latter is more metabolically active and produces more inflammation and clot-promoting compounds than does fat distributed around the periphery of the body. Fortunately, visceral fat is the first to disappear in response to exercise, a key point in

42

favor of regular exercise. The actual distribution of body fat is genetically determined, but the amount of fat stored relates directly to excess intake over output.

Obesity Genes

Obesity genes have been identified but their role is ill-defined. The overall balance between energy intake and expenditure is pretty finely tuned and only small deviations on a daily basis can produce changes in weight. A one percent excess of intake over expenditure stored as fat would produce a weight gain of 1.25 kilograms in one year. Achieving this very accurate balance depends upon an extremely complex interaction of hormones, activity, temperature exposure and other factors. The major role of hormones is that ghrelin, produced by the stomach, tells the brain it is time to eat. When food leaves the stomach another hormone, cholecystokinin, signals that the meal is over and triggers the release of other enzymes important for digestion of proteins, carbohydrates and fats.

Leptin and insulin are longer-term stabilizing factors which influence fat deposits. All of the above factors act in concert to maintain the "set point." C-75 could lower the set point. Eating too many refined carbohydrates or too much fried food can affect the delicate balance by interfering with the action of leptin and insulin on the brain. The appetite center in the hypothalamus is also affected by a number of drugs and by alcohol. Genetic variation can also push people to eat more food but obesity is by and large a behavioral problem.

VIII

The Technological Revolution

Modern humans developed between 100,000 and 150,000 years ago, coincidental with the invention of controlled agriculture. A steady and predictable source of food, which could be replenished through the seasons, led to the development of large population centers. The shift from wild meat and vegetation to cultivated grains deprived humans of many of the essential amino acids, vitamins and minerals which they have thrived on for millions of years. Although life span increased, average height diminished.

Nutritional deficiencies started to manifest themselves in skeletal remains, dental cavities developed and bacterial infections increased. Obesity, however, was not a problem. This remained the situation until approximately 100 years ago when the technological revolution led to a reduced need for hard physical labor. Improved technology has made crops of grain and dairy products both cheaper to produce and much more plentiful. Along with these changes has come the bubble of obesity which could result in a reduction in life expectation for the first time in centuries. The explosion in the prevalence of obesity is related to socioeconomic changes.

Socioeconomics and Obesity

In the U.S., wealthy people tend to be thinner than those of lower socioeconomic status. One in four adults living below the poverty line is obese; compared with one in six in the households with an income in excess of $67,000 per year. In addition, one in three African Americans is obese.

The reasons for the above are not altogether clear. It does not appear to be a simple question of eating "Krispy Kremes" instead of crispy greens. Processed foods are not just cheap, they are tasty and filling. Calorically, the best value for money is food high in refined sugar content. Lean fish or steak is much more expensive than hamburgers (Table 20).

Table 20

Socioeconomics and Obesity

- Fast foods are inexpensive, readily available, and eaten quickly
- Carbohydrate is less expensive than protein
- Eating well is expensive
- In restaurants the cheaper the food the less healthy it is
- Higher income individuals tend to be slimmer

Children, particularly, are prone to eat the wrong foods. They have some money, but not a lot and their parents are out at work. Consequently they go to the corner store and buy junk foods which they eat before the televisions on which these colorful and tasty products have been attractively advertised.

The power of advertising cannot be underestimated. One of the implications of this has been the provision of larger portions of food. In the running of a restaurant, only about twenty percent of the retail price goes toward food and therefore it is not expensive to increase the amount of food given to the consumer. Advertising super-sized meals at a bargain price is a major factor in successful marketing. Unfortunately, it results in overeating with stretching of the stomach and subsequently the desire to eat more with each meal. A vicious cycle develops so that ultimately the consumer, whether in a restaurant or at home, becomes used to taking much larger meals. Portion size increase can result in a rise in calorific intake of anything from 300 to 500 calories with each meal. Along with the bargain binge has gone a markedly increased tendency to eat in restaurants. Approximately fifty percent of food budgets are now spent in restaurants. Here, in order to make these super-sized meals more tasty and attractive, additional fats and carbohydrate are added. Unfortunately the kind of fat that is used has a high trans-fatty acid concentration. French fries, bread, pastry and salad dressing are among the items which contain trans-fatty acids.

An important factor which has led to more eating out and the consumption of more fast foods by children has been the ever-increasing tendency for both parents in a family to be engaged in fulltime employment. Under such circumstances, incomes are higher and the tendency to want to cook after a full day's work is understandably low. The result therefore has been to consume fast food.

IX

The Psychology of the Obese State

Obesity and Self-Esteem

Psychiatric problems are commonly associated with the obese state. Whether they are causative of, or consequential to, obesity may be debated. It is hardly surprising that the morbidly obese individual who cannot climb a flight of stairs, sit in a normal seat, buy or wear conventional clothes, or get on a bus or a plane, would have low self-esteem. Low self-esteem leads to social isolation, many of these obese people will not go out of the house in daylight hours. Social isolation produces depression and food provides solace to the depressed. Associated physical disorders such as sleep apnea, diabetes, hypertension and vascular disease can lead to mental changes. A psychiatrist or psychologist is an important member of the ideal management team for the obese subject.

A Behavioral Problem

It should first be said that the massively increased prevalence of obesity in the past ten years cannot be attributed to either a change in genetics or the incidence of recognizable psychiatric disorders. It is rather clearly behavioral, cultural, a submission to extrinsic pressures, such as food advertisements, and a consequence of an acquired aberration of the role and value of nutrients. Such behavioral influences may have led more people to "live to eat," rather than "eat to live." This would suggest addictive behavior, of which there may clearly be a component. Addiction to food is ostensibly more of a problem than addiction to alcohol or drugs because, difficult as the latter two are to manage, the patient may

47

temporarily be taken away from alcohol or drugs while food is an essential. Not only is food essential—we are what we eat—its accurate balance, as a need provider, may clearly be extremely difficult to control, once the regular homeostatic mechanisms fall away.

The homeostatic mechanisms that regulate eating behavior, present throughout the animal kingdom, are becoming grossly distorted in man for the first time in thousands of years. Throughout history, man has clearly suffered more from the ravages of starvation than from a plethora of food but gluttony and obesity existed with other excesses in the period of affluence of the Roman era. Although the ravages of malnutrition and the extremes of starvation in Nigeria and other African countries are depicted periodically by the media, we may have again entered an era where more suffer from excess than a shortage of food. A remarkable degree of sophistication and control goes into body weight maintenance (Table 21). The twenty-pound weight gain experienced by the average American between the ages of twenty-five and fifty-five represents a remarkably small net imbalance between energy intake and expenditure—an excess intake over expenditure of 0.3 percent of ingested calories or approximately six calories per day! (Table 22).

Table 21

Average Annual Food Intake: 1,000,000 calories

200 lb. of carbohydrate
66 lb. of fat
50 lb. of protein

Table 22

Eating an additional 1% would mean an extra 10,000 calories.
This is 1/4 cans of cola per day and will cause a gain of two lb.
  per year.
Equivalent to walking 100 miles!

Numerous biological and psychological influences may modify eating behavior. The hypothalamus and the sympathetic and

parasympathetic nervous systems, discussed above, are function-
ally influenced by psychological factors. Dietary composition per
se is not a determinant of body makeup. As both protein and
carbohydrate can be efficiently converted into fat there is no evidence that changing the relative proportions of protein, carbohydrate and fat in the diet without reducing overall caloric intake
will promote weight loss.

Psychological Factors

That psychological factors are important in governing our caloric intake is clear when we look at studies that attempt to elimi-
nate these factors. A study was carried out in which pre-weighed
bottles of milk were delivered to the houses of thirty-seven babies.
The bottles were then collected for re-weighing and the determina-
tion of food intake. By varying the dilution of the milk, different
energy densities, of which the mothers were unaware, were given
at different times. The babies fed with half-strength milk increased
their volume intake by 80 percent but not 100 percent. This would
suggest that appetite may be related to volume rather than energy
intake. Later in life individual food preferences would make such
a study impossible.

Studies in older malnourished children in Jamaica, however,
demonstrated the development of a voracious appetite after long-
term food deprivation. This might be an explanation for the often
observed rapid weight gain which follows a period of dieting.
Outside of infancy, psychological factors soon impose a considerable influence on dietary intake, which is affected by the color,
texture, smell, taste and energy content of food. Studies have
shown that the individual's selection of food reflects a response to
food availability and palatability, rather than energy content, hence
the effect of fast foods on weight. Such factors are social as well
as psychological. The situation is complex in that animals may
vary their food intake in order to obtain sufficient amounts of
essential minerals or vitamins when food concentrations of the
latter are low. If such instincts ever existed in man they have now
probably been lost.

Society & Eating Habits

Societies, across the nations, have developed an antagonistic attitude toward obesity. Obese children tend to be disliked, looked down upon and regarded as figures of fun. Their obese state is associated with shame as they are thought to be self indulgent and lacking in will power. By contrast, the obese children are regarded as being responsible for their condition, whereas disabled children are not, and the latter receive sympathy and support. The feeding of babies and children has substantial emotional overtones and the provision of food may be associated with signs of affection. Obese parents tend to beget or create obese children. The availability and palatability of food influences intake. High caloric value of food tends to equate with palatability and foods high in sugar content tend to be more available by being cheaper than more ideal foods.

Social and family pressures can lead to overeating, as it is often regarded as a sign of appreciation to eat as much as possible of the food presented. We spend so much time sitting around the table eating. Important life events such as birthdays, successes, marriages and even funerals are celebrated by feasts. Such practices are not new. The Romans derived great pleasure from eating and often overate in a gluttonous fashion. "Ear ticklers" existed in Roman times, people who were skilled at rubbing the ears of those who had overeaten, only to induce vomiting and thereby enable the party goer to begin eating again. The mechanism of this procedure was that the vagus nerve or "wandering" nerve supplies not only the stomach but has branches to the external ear. Stimulation of the ear activates the vagus nerve and can produce contractions of the stomach which induces vomiting.

The Ritual of Eating

The eating of food becomes an important ritual. We all like good foods, a variety of foods and we not only socialize around the table but we hold business meetings as well. If indeed food becomes an addiction, which is the case in some morbidly obese individuals, then it is one with which the addicted must constantly contend, as food is not only essential but is around us always.

50

Diets eaten in different countries vary very widely but most nations have, over the centuries, developed diets which, though widely differing in their content, maintain the body in good functional health without any marked nutritional deficiencies. Recently, studies have shown that Puerto Rican women living in the Continental U.S. increase weight with both the longer period they have spent there and the better their English. This is persuasive evidence that social factors rather than genetic ones are important.

Obesity and Depression

Though perhaps difficult accurately to categorize, the psychological factors which pertain to the obese state are significant and considerable. The higher the body/mass index, the greater is the incidence of depression. A number of factors contribute to the development of psychological problems which culminate in chronic depression. Discrimination leads to low self-worth and a reduced quality of life. Family and sexual relationships suffer and problems frequently arise in the workplace. Employment can be difficult to obtain. Over two-thirds of obese patients report abuse, physical in 34 percent, sexual in 12 percent and psychological in 64 percent. One third of morbidly obese patients report a family history of alcoholism. Conversely alcoholism is rare in the morbidly obese subject.

Body Image and the Psyche

Body image is an aspect of overall self-image. A woman who was sexually abused in childhood may use her size as a protection against attracting men. Despite her desire to lose weight, she may get more and more anxious as she becomes more shapely. Another person, who equates food with love, or weight with power, will experience much inner conflict about changing his or her lifestyle when losing weight.

To be successful, all psychotherapy must address emotional dysregulation, impulsive behavior and cognitive/perceptual distortions. Group and individual therapy, particularly cognitive-behavioral therapy, can highlight rationalizations, reframe negative patterns of thinking and provide a more realistic manner of self-assessment. A recognition of one's own mental functioning, and how one solves problems is essential to reshape those attitudes from the past which may sabotage dieting efforts.

Fatness Was Equated with Success

Early in the twentieth century, when tuberculosis and other infectious diseases were still rampant, to be thin was often perceived as a sign of sickness, poverty or neglect. The prize of every family was plump "healthy" children; the plump female was "womanly"; the plump male, watch chain stretched across his belly, looked "prosperous." Most people had heard of calories and knew that sweets were fattening, but paid little or no attention to the caloric contents of what they ate.

When World War II brought rationing, meat and butter became luxury items. Gas was rationed, people walked, yet most middle-aged adults in the U.S. were overweight, and few exercised for health. It was expected that a woman would lose her "figure" after thirty, and have to wear a girdle. Men padded their shoulders and wore double breasted suits to hide middle-aged bellies. "Old" was synonymous with "fat," and nobody thought anything could be done about it.

The Impact of Television

After the war, the biggest change in American life was due to television. TV changed the eating habits of America, but not for the better. The "TV dinner" predominated on the American menu, as everyone gathered around the new center of the home. TV's advertising potential was quickly realized and exploited by the food industry, telling children to eat more sugared cereals and tempting adults to indulge in "double" cheeseburgers, chips, and malts and multiple snacks.

Advertising of Food

Advertising showed America the face it wanted to see—big, affluent and carefree, untouched by war or want. Cars were oversized, sporting big fins and capacious seats. In the new supermarkets, myriad food packages promised "more" for your money. Restaurants served big steaks on bigger plates, along with the new, huge, "salad bar." Truly, only too much was enough. It is no wonder indeed that Americans learned to overeat, long before the crisis of today.

Psychological Aspects Related to Exercise

Lack of exercise is an important factor in the obesity equation. It has been shown that the less walking a person does in his day-to-day activities the more likely he is to be overweight. Exercise increases academic performance, assertiveness, confidence, emotional stability, independence, memory, mood, sexual satisfaction and well-being. In addition exercise programs decrease absenteeism, anger, anxiety, depression and even alcohol abuse. Obese subjects are often opposed to exercise programs. They are self-conscious and frequently have difficulty in performing the exercises because they are carrying so much extra weight or they may be restricted by joint pains or breathlessness. Many morbidly obese patients are too disabled to exercise, or even to climb a flight of stairs. Those who can exercise are frequently discouraged by the slow results achieved from exercise programs and the fact that a can of cola contains all of the calories expended in a thirty-minute exercise schedule!

The importance of exercise can not be overemphasized. Exercise is important from the point of view of preventing heart attacks, strokes and the development of diabetes. The benefits of exercise are clearly visible by increased muscle mass and often increased activity and alertness. Exercise does not necessarily increase hunger. In fact, a thirty-to-forty minute walk produces well-being by virtue of an endorphin drive and can lead to a suppression of appetite. Also, the results of participating in an exercise program are a disincentive for the subject then to go home and eat excessive amounts of food.

Exercise not only burns calories in itself, but tends to increase basal metabolic rate, giving rise to a further erosion on the calorific load. Another useful manifestation of exercise is that it stimulates muscle production and converts fat into muscle. Finally the endorphin drive produced by exercise results in a feeling of well-being and enables people to adopt a more positive attitude toward life and its problems.

Eating Disorders

Once viewed as disorders of choice alone, eating disorders have been shown to have polygenetic factors in common with each other as well as sharing risk factors with many psychiatric illnesses. Family and twin studies suggest that eating disorders run in families and are due to addictive genetic influences which affect food intake and body weight. Neuropeptides within the brain interact with gut-related peptides in a complex pattern influencing appetite, the after-meal satiety point, and long term body weight homeostasis.

Genetically susceptible obese persons may not respond normally to biological signals. Neuroimaging studies are now being used to study brain reaction patterns to pictures, smells, tastes and ideas in obese and normal weight persons. One such project by nutritional researchers studied the PET scans of matched groups of obese and normal weight men after consuming a tasty snack following a fast. The obese men had significantly greater regional blood flow in the emotional and impulsiveness areas of the brain than the normal-weight men. This raises the question of whether obese persons have a qualitatively different taste response and decision making pathway, a brain reward system particularly sensitive to food, which reinforces their eating patterns by intensifying their brain reward responses?

The three major eating disorders are (1) anorexia nervosa (food restricting); (2) bulimia nervosa (binging and purging); and (3) binge eating disorder (binging only). In anorexia nervosa and bulimia nervosa, subjects are preoccupied with their body shape and size. They are terrified of being fat. They binge and purge, using self-induced vomiting, laxatives or excessive exercise to compensate for their loss of eating control. Those with anorexia nervosa have a delusional belief that they are fat, when they are actually emaciated. Those with bulimia nervosa fear becoming fat or getting fatter.

Worldwide twin studies showed that the inheritability of bulimia nervosa is between 50 percent and 83 percent. Environmental factors are less important and that the liability for developing bulimia nervosa is predominantly dependent on genetic factors. The remainder of the risk of developing bulimia nervosa comes out of unique environmental factors or special stressors one may encounter. Anorexia nervosa is also a mainly genetic disorder in which inheritability is 58 percent–76 percent. Anorexia nervosa and bulimia nervosa share related personality phenotypes, such as perfectionism, body dissatisfaction and a drive for thinness.

Binge Eating Disorder

Binging is eating a much larger amount of food than normal in a short time, usually less than two hours. Binging is a factor in all of the eating disorders. What sets Binge Eating Disorder apart from others is the lack of purging, and the high frequency of binging, two more times weekly.

The triggers to binge are extremely mood sensitive, susceptible to hormonal changes, fatigue, life events, disappointments with oneself or with others. Bingers may feel a binge "coming on" and gather foods in advance, or may just eat whatever is at hand, even food they don't ordinarily like. Bingers usually eat alone at home, to hide the amount or types of food consumed, but they may also begin at a party or restaurant and continue at home. The key feature is, once started, the binger feels out of control, compelled to keep eating to the point of discomfort and even of misery. Each bout leaves the binger feeling ashamed and disgusted, but unable to stop doing it again and again. This leads to a chronic feeling of guilt and dread of discovery—addictive behavior.

Food Cravings and Binge Eating

Food cravings have a continuously disruptive effect on attempts to diet and constitute a continuous goad to binge eating behavior. Researchers have been teasing out the difference between craving, needing, and liking certain foods, independent of hunger. Virtually 100 percent of young women and 70 percent of young men have experienced food cravings during the past year. Contrary to popular opinion, a craving is not in response to a body deficit of nutrients or calories.

In a prospective study of craving, participants were given a vanilla nutrition supplement drink as their total food for five days. If the participants lost weight they were dropped from the study. Frequency of food cravings before the study was compared with food cravings during the study and during a recovery period, when participants could eat whatever they wanted. A normal control group ate as usual and were also given frequent samples of the vanilla drink. On the monotonous diet, food cravings peaked on the second day in all subjects. Under MRI brain scan, subjects were asked to imagine their favorite food for thirty seconds, then the vanilla nutrition drink for thirty seconds. Every participant showed MRI patterns of cravings during imagining their favorite food, and none did while imagining the vanilla nutrition drink. The monotonous diet group had significantly more cravings than the normal diet group. This showed up in three craving-specific areas if the brain, the hippocampus, the insula and the caudate nucleus. The same brain pathways may also be involved in feeding, not just in craving.

Food cravings, alcohol and drug cravings all use the same brain pathways. The image of food or drugs evokes more intense reactions than the substance itself. This suggests the powerful role of habit is reinforcing these biologically bound food cravings. The same pattern of increased craving is clearly demonstrated when a person attempts to stop smoking, another area where habits and cravings strongly overlap. Even after stopping, the former smoker may experience cravings when presented with any smoking related situation or memory. So too, certain life situations may bring on a food craving.

Binge Eating and Other Psychiatric Disorders

Obese persons with binge eating disorder have higher lifetime episodes of depression, panic disorder, generalized anxiety disorders and bulimia than subjects without binge eating disorder. Those with binge eating behavior also show significantly higher rates of major depression, posttraumatic stress disorder, phobias and alcohol dependency than non-bingers. Not surprisingly, this population has increased rates of medical comorbidities than non-bingers.

Other psychiatric conditions also are characterized in part by binging or increased eating. Bulimia is common in major depressive disorders and atypical depressions. In atypical depression a person eats too much and sleeps too much. Women are far more likely to have this form of depression than men. Most depressed men actually lose weight during a depressive episode.

Those with schizophrenia, schizo-affective disorder and bipolar (manic depressive) disorder have high rates of overweight and obesity. In bipolar disorder, patients suffer almost twice as much obesity as in the general population. Anti-psychotic and other medications may compound the problem for these individuals by causing increased eating and weight gain over long periods of time. Those with mental retardation also have higher rates of overweight and obesity. They may not be able to regulate their own caloric intake for personal or environmental reasons.

In females, major depression during childhood is associated with obesity. The longer the depression, the more obese the adults become. Childhood abuse, sexual, physical and verbal, also may lead to an increased tendency toward overweight and obesity in adulthood, particularly in women. Childhood abuse can permanently alter a person's brain and adrenal gland reactions to stressful situations, which can lead to altered eating patterns.

Treatment

Obesity has only recently been declared to be a medical disorder in its own right. Treatment options for obesity encompass medications, various types of psychotherapy, and surgery. All plans are based on proper diet and exercise as a life course. As this overview shows, the variety of social and genetic variables in each person who seeks treatment will necessitate specific treatments and a long-term commitment to weight normalization, using all appropriate means.

To be successful, all psychotherapy must address emotional dysregulation, impulsive behavior and cognitive/perceptual distortions. The latter includes body image and self-esteem issues, as well as anxieties which lead to impulsive eating. Group and individual therapy, particularly cognitive-behavioral therapy, can highlight rationalizations, reframe negative patterns of thinking and provide a more realistic manner of self-assessment. A recognition of one's own mental functioning, and how one solves problems, is essential to change.

Antidepressants and mood-stabilizing medications are extremely useful in aiding mood regulation, and dealing with craving and compulsive eating. Appetite suppressants may need to be used long-term as well. Surgical treatment must have extensive medical follow-up and psychiatric and nutritional support. This calls for a high level of commitment by the patient to a permanent life change, with a realistic timetable and a clear set of expectations and personal responsibilities worked out with the treatment team.

Understanding obesity as a medical disorder calls for seeing it as a dynamic pathological body state, arising from a convergence of genetic susceptibilities, and sustained by sociocultural and environmental influences on eating habits. Widely held prejudices against obese persons as lazy or morally weak should be confronted by all parties and dealt with openly, to change medical as well as social attitudes. Public funding of preventive measures could begin a campaign of national awareness to stem this serious epidemic and its many consequences, on a personal and a national level.

X

Physical Activity and Body Weight

The importance of energy expenditure has already been stressed, and this remains a fundamental issue in considering weight stability. Physical inactivity is a major factor in the present day weight problem that afflicts so many American citizens (Table 23). Individuals vary widely in terms of their energy expenditure as a result of their differing physical activity. While increasing numbers run marathons, greater numbers refrain from indulging in any form of physical activity at all. Physical energy expenditure ranges from static physical exercise such as rapidly increasing and decreasing muscle tone and gesticulating, to voluntarily moving in athletic activity, as in running.

The energy expenditure of minimal daily activity in a non-exercising person is about 50 percent greater than the basal metabolic rate, the latter being the amount of expenditure required to maintain the stability of the individual while totally resting, such as lying in bed. Moderately active individuals add approximately another 20 percent to this figure. Obesity in itself, once established, limits physical activity and prohibits most forms of athletics. Females tend to expend fewer calories by physical activity than do males. Females with their smaller muscular mass may find moving their excess weight more difficult than obese males, and alter their pattern of activity accordingly. It has also been suggested that obese individuals are likely to show a reduced variety of fine movements, such as moving around in a chair and gesticulating, than those of normal weight (Table 24).

Table 23

Exercise

Exercise is good.
Weight training is better!
Select a regime you can comply with.
Don't overdo it to begin with.
Walking is excellent.

Table 24

Energy Expenditure and Exercise

Day-to-day normal activities	500–1,000 calories
Walking	300 cal/hr
Cycling	400 cal/hr
Running	500–600 cal/hr
Rowing	600 cal/hr
Swimming	400–600 cal/hr

Studies comparing the body composition in heavy and light workers show that these groups have similar fat content and clearly those engaged in light work should modify their food intake to maintain the same sort of equilibrium as the heavy worker. The effects of physical exercise in relation to total energy turnover each day are relatively small. However, it has been shown that those who walk more, weigh less. Furthermore, the decline in physical activity in the population as a whole probably contributes to the increased prevalence of obesity. The exact mechanism is not fully understood. Whatever the cause of obesity, it can be argued that increased physical activity is a useful aid to weight reduction and to maintaining the reduced body weight.

Exercise Programs

It is usually necessary to walk for in excess of thirty minutes a day to establish any significant weight loss. Unfortunately, of those beginning a heavy exercise program involving thirty minutes or more of exercise daily, fewer than 30 percent will persist for any significant length of time. Most studies placing emphasis on exercise programs have shown a very high attrition rate even when these trials last only a few weeks or months. More intense forms of exercise than walking, such as jogging, are more likely to result in a lack of compliance. Losing weight by exercise therefore depends considerably upon the motivation of the individual. The increase in work output would seem to affect total energy turnover to only a small extent.

It is possible that the decrease in activity that occurs with age may form the basis for the decline in muscle mass and lean body mass as people grow older. Replacement of lean tissue by fat associated with aging worsens the problem of energy imbalance, since the basal need for energy falls with the total reduction in metabolically active lean tissue; this will lead to a further drop in the basal metabolic rate and a tendency to gain body fat. It should be emphasized to all of those entering weight-reduction programs that the physiological beneficial effects of short periods of moderately intense exercise are well documented and that a minimum of twenty minutes of moderate activity three times per week is good for the cardiovascular system. This degree of activity also seems to play an important role in improving an individual's sense of well-being, probably by the production of endorphins. It is unclear whether this amount of exercise helps to maintain lean body mass. Not only are the effects of aerobic exercise positive, but working with weights increases the ratio of body protein to body fat which is beneficial and this also stimulates metabolic activity. Exercise is also good for the brain!

XI
Nutritional Facts and Figures

Depending upon size, age, and activity level an adult woman typically needs about 1,700–2,000 calories per day; the typical adult man needs 2,000–2,500 calories. With increasing age, calorific requirements fall. To lose one pound of fat in a week, a person needs to reduce his caloric intake by 3,500 calories or the approximately equivalent of two days of food—it's tough! To lose fat, one should not concentrate on eating less fat per se. It is the total caloric intake that adds weight and easily taken carbohydrates produce as much weight gain in pounds of fat as does fat itself. It's not just a question of eating less calories, though. An adequate diet must contain essential vitamins and minerals as well, though these can be covered by over-the-counter medications available at pharmacies and health food stores.

Cholesterol

Cholesterol is a waxy lipid that is an essential constituent of every cell in the body. It is manufactured in the liver as well as being ingested. Lipoproteins carry cholesterol from the liver through the body via the bloodstream. As mentioned earlier bad cholesterol is low-density-lipoprotein (LDL) which contributes to cardiac and vascular disease. High-density lipoprotein (HDL) "sweeps up" some of the cholesterol deposits and is therefore regarded as good cholesterol. High levels of LDL-cholesterol lead to heart disease but avoiding foods which are high in cholesterol does not necessarily decrease the amount of cholesterol in the blood. Saturated fats used to be thought to be the main culprit underlying vascular disease. These fats which are present in dairy products raise high-density lipoproteins as well as low-density lipoproteins so that a balance is maintained. Another type of fat, transfats, are partially hydrogenated vegetable oils, which increase LDL cholesterol and decrease HDL cholesterol. This causes the depositing of cholesterol on blood vessels without the "mopping up" factor of HDL cholesterol being present (Figure 4). Trans fats are present in large amounts in fried foods, chips, cookies and cakes. These substances, in themselves, contain no cholesterol but they stimulate cholesterol production by the liver.

Refined Carbohydrates

Fat, however, is not the real enemy. Eating fat does not make you fat, conversely it can help you to eat less overall. Refined carbohydrates, which cause the blood sugar to shoot up rapidly, are the main enemy. Not all carbohydrates are bad. Many vegetables and fruits are high in vitamins and minerals. They also contain antioxidants which dispose of potentially harmful oxygen byproducts called free radicals. These substances also contain fiber, which can lower cholesterol and stabilize blood sugar levels. In giving dietary advice, therefore, one should recommend a strategy of eating in moderation and avoiding trans fats and refined carbohydrates. Instead, eat foods which are minimally processed such as brown rice, blueberries and fish sautéed with garlic in olive oil.

Meats

In preparing meat, external fat should be removed. Portions should be restricted to the size of the palm of the hand. Expensive cuts of beef taste better because they contain more fat! Veal is low in fat but high in cholesterol. Lamb and pork tend to contain a lot of fat. Cutting the fat from pork leaves healthy lean meat. Bacon is high in sodium and in fat and sausages are high in carbohydrates and fat.

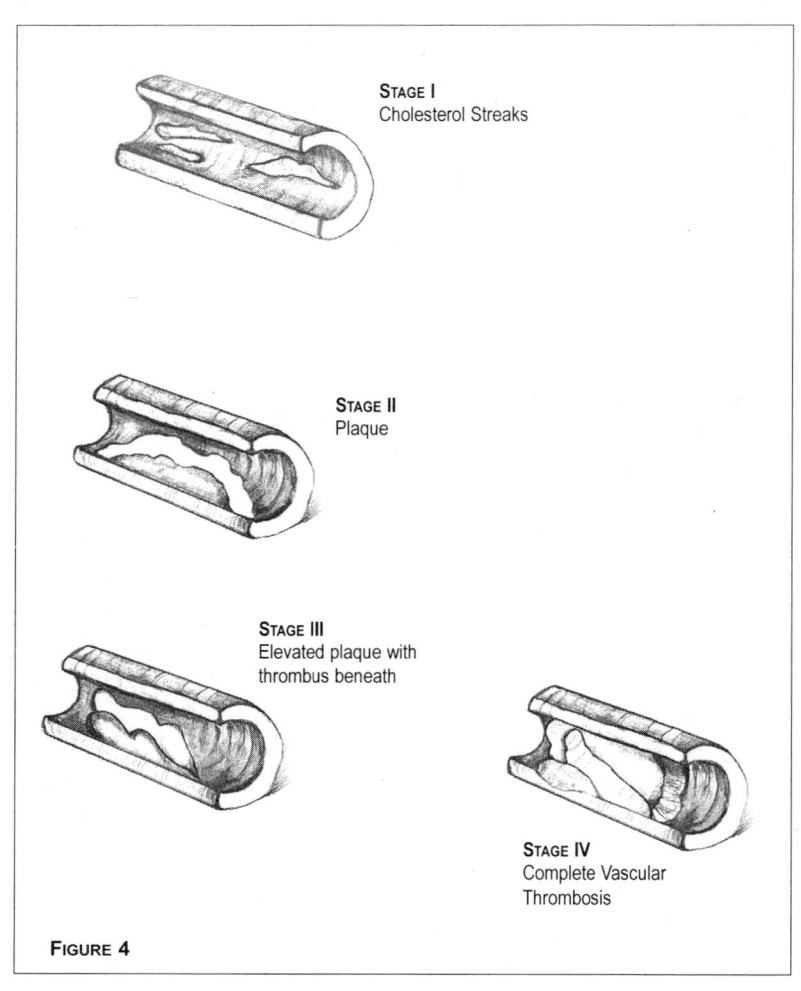

STAGE I
Cholesterol Streaks

STAGE II
Plaque

STAGE III
Elevated plaque with
thrombus beneath

STAGE IV
Complete Vascular
Thrombosis

FIGURE 4

The development of arteriosclerosis

Fish

Fish, particularly salmon, mackerel and sardines, are an excellent source of omega-3 fatty acids. Fish are rich in calcium. Farm-raised salmon and tuna may accumulate high levels of mercury and other toxins. It is safer to eat wild salmon rather than the now-ubiquitous farm-raised salmon. Batter-dipped white fish are high in fat, particularly the trans fats. Shellfish are high in cholesterol but low in calories; the cholesterol is not usually significant enough to boost levels in the bloodstream.

Chicken

High in protein, low in fat and cholesterol, chicken, without the skin, makes for healthy eating. Turkey is the leanest meat of all and with the skin removed the fat content of turkey breast is less than 1 percent. Duck, from which the skin is removed is, contrary to popular belief, low in fat. Game birds, such as pheasant, are very low in fat.

Wild game, like deer, are a good source of protein, which is also low in fat.

Dairy Products

Milk contains calcium, protein, zinc and the fat-soluble vitamins. Cheese is similar to milk. Eggs are high in cholesterol though the whites are an excellent source of protein and the yolks are not necessarily bad. Yogurt is good but tends to be sweetened with refined sugar. Bacon, eggs and sausage fried in butter are not a healthy combination of food stuffs. Margarines, which are free of trans fat and contain twice as much polyunsaturated as saturated fat, are a healthy source of fat. Vegetable oils are good, they contain large amounts of heart-healthy omega-3 and omega-6 fatty acids.

Other Foods

Nuts contain a large amount of fat but also many beneficial nutrients such as the B-vitamins. They are good in small amounts.

Coconuts are high in phytosterols, compounds that have been shown to reduce levels of blood cholesterol. They are however also high in saturated fat and carbohydrate but contain no cholesterol.

Vital nutrients are plentiful in seeds which also contain fiber and frequently omega-3 fatty acids. Flax seeds are particularly high in omega-3 fatty acids and have anticoagulant properties. They may also be useful in treating some tumors.

Soy protein is the only complete vegetable protein which contains all of the essential amino acids. Soy also contains iron, calcium, magnesium, vitamin E, riboflavin, thiamin, folate and good fats. Soy flour is higher in protein and lower in carbohydrate than wheat flour and it lacks gluten. Legumes are low in fat and contain no cholesterol. They are rich in minerals and fiber. Hummus contains a high concentration of fat.

Cereals

Bread is high in calories and carbohydrate. Croissants are the most calorie dense. A bagel can contain 400 calories. Whole wheat bread is the lowest in calories and highest in fiber. Muffins need not be so calorie dense, but contain trans fatty acids. Pasta is low in fat and cholesterol, but high in carbohydrate. Rice is rich in carbohydrates, low in fat and cholesterol and a good source of B-vitamins. Whole grains are digested slowly and therefore they don't produce rapid rises in blood glucose levels. Most cereals are a rich source of carbohydrates, other nutrients may be added. Of all the cereal grains and grasses, oats are the most nutritious. They provide more protein than rice and they contain B-vitamins, iron, selenium and fiber.

Fruit and Vegetables

Fruits and vegetables are important to the healthy diet. They are rich in antioxidants and contain vitamins, minerals and fiber.

Highest in antioxidants are blueberries and blue, red and purple berries are high in anthocyanins. The most healthy of all the vegetables is asparagus. Carrots are rich in vitamin A. Onions and garlic are helpful in preventing thrombosis in vessels.

Fast Food

Probably the biggest contemporary problem which afflicts us in relation to obesity is the social trend, or compulsion, to eat in fast food restaurants or take-outs. A single meal of a super burger, jumbo fries, mega soda and fried pie greatly exceeds the daily recommended caloric requirements and is high in sodium but deficient in vitamins and minerals. Just the "beef" part of a double burger contains 580 calories with 33 grams of fat and 47 grams of carbohydrate. Whether purchased from McDonald's or Burger King, the calorific counts are similar.

Kentucky Fried Chicken contains a large amount of fat in the batter and in the skin. An "Extra Crispy Breast" contains 470 calories and a "Chunky Chicken Pot Pie" exudes 770 calories. Taco Bell's products tend to be lower in cholesterol but a taco salad with shell (crust) contains a staggering 800 calories! This makes the taco salad higher in saturated fat calories, carbohydrates and sodium than a "Big Mac" or a "Whopper."

The health message as far as pizza is concerned is "go for the thinnest crust, least cheese and most vegetables." One slice of "Beef, Personal Plan" at Pizza Hut contains 710 calories. Veggie pizzas on a thin crust are probably the best, but pizzas do not create healthy eating.

XII
Nutrition and Metabolism

Under resting conditions a normal healthy adult male burns approximately ten calories per pound per day. With normal activity this caloric requirement virtually doubles. The caloric requirement is met by the use of the three main food stuffs, carbohydrates, fats and proteins. The body initially burns the carbohydrates, glucose and glycogen, but body stores contain little of these and therefore fasting will lead to fat and protein being burned. The basic requirement of living cells is to use protein for repair and replacement of cells and to supply the energy to drive these reactions. In order to fuel the required metabolic activities the body needs to generate a substance, adenosine triphosphate (ATP).

Carbohydrate Metabolism

The gut rapidly breaks down complex sugars into simple ones, predominately glucose, fructose and galactose. Sugars are absorbed through the small intestine and transported to the liver. Some of the glucose remains in the circulation to maintain the blood sugar at a constant level. It is transported to cells to provide energy. Glucose is broken down in the cells by a process known as glycolysis which requires oxygen.

Fat Metabolism

About 40 percent of calories in the average American diet are derived from fat. Fats and oils are triesters of glycerol and various fatty acids. The ability of lipids to be stored in the body as fat provides the source for continuous energy production. Fats are used once carbohydrate stores have been metabolized which is usually after a period of about twelve hours of starvation. Absorption of lipids depends upon their being mixed with bile and then they are absorbed in the small intestine, and converted into triglycerides which are transported via the lymphatic system or directly into the blood stream. Fat is not only stored but is used to form an essential constituent of cell membranes. A reduction in carbohydrate intake causes an increase in the breakdown of triglycerides and free fatty acids.

Virtually all tissues, except the brain, require lipids as an energy source. When excessive amounts of lipids are metabolized and used for energy, breakdown products, (which accumulate in the bloodstream) such as aceto acetic acid, give rise to a condition known as ketosis. Criticism of the Atkins diet is that it has led to production of ketosis.

Protein Metabolism

The main function of protein is to provide the building blocks for cells. Proteins can be utilized as a fuel source for energy in times of stress. Protein molecules taken in the diet are broken down by digestive enzymes into peptides and amino acids. These are the basic constituents of all larger protein molecules. There is a high turnover of body protein and many grams of protein are carried throughout the body per hour. The constituent products of protein, amino acids are linked to cellular proteins and stored as protein. Once the cell is replete, unused excess amino acids are converted to keto acids. A breakdown product of amino acids is ammonia, which in large amounts is toxic and depresses brain function. Protein is essential for the production of the nucleic acids, DNA and RNA, which are the key to the fundamental genetic structure of man.

Nutritional Requirements

Nutritional requirements vary with age, sex, and body size and can be influenced by drugs, hormones and disease states. Carbohydrates provide approximately half the human energy requirement. They may be ingested as simple sugars or more complex carbohydrates. Certain tissues such as the brain, blood cells and the kidney have an obligatory requirement for glucose.

Lipids, as well as being a source of energy, play an important role in the structure and function of cells.

Proteins, unlike carbohydrates and lipids, are not held in storage. They do, however, make up approximately twenty percent of the lean body mass as muscle. Proteins exist in the form of enzymes, which are required to enable chemical reactions to be carried out inside the body. Another important role of proteins is to provide a source of essential amino acids. These are amino acids which are needed for normal body function, but cannot be produced by the body. Dietary proteins contain these essential amino acids in varying concentrations.

Many of the normal chemical processes essential for life require vitamins. Deficiencies in these vitamins cause well-defined diseases. A total of thirteen vitamins have been identified as being essential in human nutrition. Five of these are fat soluble and eight are water soluble. Fat soluble vitamins are: A, D, E and K. Vitamins A, C, and E, together with the mineral selenium are anti-oxidants, important in breakdown of free radical oxidation products. Deficiencies of individual vitamins produce well-known syndromes. One which is well known to the public is scurvy, which historically used to be common on long sea voyages. Scurvy, which presents with bleeding from the gums, is due to a deficiency in vitamin C or ascorbic acid. On long transatlantic sea voyages, sailors became deficient in vitamin C and developed a full-blown syndrome of scurvy, which ultimately became treatable by the provision of limes to sailors embarking on such long voyages.

In addition to vitamins, there are nineteen minerals and trace minerals which are essential to humans, and they may be grouped into four categories based on their function. Calcium, phosphorus, magnesium and zinc are structural components of bone. A second group, sodium, potassium and chloride, function as major charged ions within the cellular mechanism. Calcium and magnesium are both structural components of bone and function as charged ions. Trace minerals which are necessary for normal health include iron, zinc, copper, selenium, manganese, molybdenum, cobalt, iodine and chromium.

Minerals are necessary to prevent deficiency states and the intake of minerals can be low even in the obese, but particularly so following surgery for morbid obesity. Malabsorption, the consequences of a number of diseases and the effects of some drugs can alter mineral balances.

Calcium is the most abundant mineral in the body and plays a vital role in muscular and cardiac activity. It is also involved in coagulation of the blood, and the secretion of certain hormones. Excessive intakes of Vitamins A and D can give rise to high levels of calcium. Low levels of calcium may be associated with low levels of albumin and magnesium. Magnesium is an important mineral within the cells and is involved in many chemical reactions. Levels of magnesium frequently fall following obesity surgery. Conversely, too much magnesium can cause cell damage and renal failure. Trace elements also tend to be depleted after obesity surgery. A common manifestation of zinc deficiency is hair loss. This usually responds promptly to replacement of the missing zinc. Iron levels may also suffer and in association with this, anemia may develop.

Assessment of Nutritional State

The body mass index, weight in kilograms over height in meters^2, is sometimes referred to Quetelet's Index. A Quetelet's Index of twenty to twenty-five is associated with a minimal risk of mortality. Once the obese range is entered, mortality increases markedly with increasing weight. Numerous methods have been developed to estimate the amount of fatty tissue in the human body. The simplest of these uses the anthropometric technique of skin fold thickness. The triceps skin fold is most commonly used. Here the skin and underlying tissues superficial to the triceps muscle at the back of the upper arm is pinched together and the thickness of the skin fold is measured. The fat thickness is also measured over other muscles in the body, in particular over the shoulders, abdomen and thighs. These skin fold thicknesses are compared with those expressed in tables for differing degrees of obesity.

Skeletal muscle can be estimated by using another anthropometric technique that of mid-arm circumference. This is the measurement of lean arm tissue, which is then compared with existing standards. The mid-arm circumference is calculated by subtracting the mid-arm fat circumference from the mid-arm circumference using a mathematical formula. More sophisticated methods of measuring body fat include densitromity, which involves the patient being submerged in water, and imaging techniques such as computerized tomography and ultrasound. Electrical conductivity or impedance measurements can also be used to estimate body fat and are based on the difference in conductivity of lean and fat tissue.

XIII

Conservative Methods of Treating Obesity

Unsupervised Methods and Recognized Diets

It has been estimated that, at any one time, two-thirds of women and one-third of men are trying to lose weight. Over one-third of the population are regular users of one or more slimming products, most of which are specifically advertised as helping weight-loss and are available in the general marketplace. Overall, most attempted slimming is self-administered and self-controlled without supervision. There are, however, no authoritative guidelines for health education of the general public regarding the optimal type of diet.

Over-the-Counter Diets

A wide variety of methods are therefore in use for unsupervised slimming (Table 25). Women's magazines and even special magazines devoted to the subject exist in large numbers. Industry also produces "slimmers" breads and crisp breads and also low-energy soft drinks. Over-the-counter items such as methyl-cellulose-based products, which are deemed to reduce hunger by providing bulk to fill the stomach, are widely available. However, there is no scientific evidence that these are of any value in reducing food intake or producing weight loss. Another recommended strategy is to take a glucose load of fifty grams ten to twenty minutes before a meal and this, it is claimed, reduces subsequent food intake.

Table 25

Unsupervised?

Sources:
  Magazines
  Newspapers
  Television
  Internet
  Often crash diets

Calorie-counted meals are widely available in supermarkets, but there is no evidence that they can be relied upon as a vehicle for long-term weight loss.

Organizations and magazines run self-help groups. The magazines give substantive advice on slimming, but often perpetrate incorrect nutritional principles. They frequently advocate "crash diets," which almost invariably lead to a rebound weight gain, or they focus on specific food stuffs which may be inappropriate for long-term strategy in achieving weight loss.

Historically, diets have focused on reduced fat intake. For over half a century, emphasis has been placed, by the medical profession, on lowering cholesterol and reducing the intake of animal fat and dairy products. Fat contains nine calories per gram as opposed to four calories per gram for carbohydrate and protein, but fat is not so easily eaten in large amounts as is carbohydrate, and carbohydrate excesses are converted into fat.

Successful slimming clearly depends on a number of factors, many of which are not appreciated, but the subject's ability to keep to a particular dietary scheme is as important as the total energy intake. Many individuals find it difficult to sustain any regime for a prolonged period of time and some diets may be complicated and expensive to produce. Furthermore individual's energy requirements vary considerably so that results achieved by specific diets can be different (Table 26).

Table 26

Diets

Over the Counter
Methyl Cellulose—swells in the stomach—no value
No-calorie diet soda—use these
Magazines and diet books—no proven value

Named Diets

Low Fat	Ornish
(Fat is nine calories per gram)	
Low Carbohydrate	Atkins
(Carbohydrate is four calories	
per gram)	Sugar Busters
	South Beach

Calorie-counting Diets

On most calorie-counting diets the subject is allowed to eat any foods that cumulatively provide a given energy intake. Although there is freedom of choice, there are many disadvantages. Food needs to be weighed precisely, and energy intake is calculated from this. Commonly patients will state that these diets fail when, in reality, it is unlikely that the patient is adhering to the diet. A slight variation on this theme is the "set diet" in which a diet sheet provides the week's menu for three meals per day. These menus offer variety and alternatives are frequently given (Table 27).

Table 27

Eating an additional 1 percent would mean an extra 10,000 calories per year.
This is $1\frac{1}{4}$ cans of cola per day and will cause a gain of 2 lb. per year.
Equivalent to walking 100 miles!

Lowfat Diets

With lowfat diets, the individual is provided with a list of foods which are high in fat and which must be avoided or severely restricted. These diets often originated specifically to reduce cholesterol levels and thereby reduce the risk of heart disease. Carbohydrates are not usually specifically restricted with these diets, which are prone to fail.

Low Carbohydrate Diets

Diets which are low in carbohydrate actually go back a long way. Banting, who discovered insulin over a century ago, devised low-carbohydrate diets for treating diabetes. While these have continued to be used, emphasis has only recently been placed on them as a major strategy for weight loss. Those most widely used are the Atkins Diet, Sugar Busters and the South Beach Diet.

The Atkins Diet

The Atkins diet, as claimed by the late author, is an easy to stay with regime that combines nutrition and vitranutrient supplements into a unique, not only weight reducing, but also age-defying program. Atkins claims that this diet adds many years to life; boosts immune defenses; enhances brain function and memory; reduces the risk of cardiovascular disease, permits weight loss without calorie restriction and combats adult-onset diabetes (Table 32).

Atkins promulgated this diet against strong opposition from august bodies such as the American Cardiological Society.

The Atkins diet involves a radical reduction of intake of carbohydrates. Those carbohydrates which are allowed are complex and unrefined, basically starchy foods including whole grains and lentils. Table sugar, sweets, cakes, cookies and soft drinks are banned. These latter foods have a very high glycemic index that sends insulin levels soaring. Simple carbohydrates should be no more than about 3 percent of the total diet. Pasta, bread, white rice, baked goods, candy and sodas are forbidden.

Simple sugars are rapidly digested as they "bump up" the blood sugar, producing a rapid outpouring of large amounts of insulin from the pancreas. This causes the glucose to fall and creates a craving for more carbohydrates. As insulin resistance develops the excess sugar accumulates in the blood producing the effects of diabetes.

This situation also leads to obesity as the excess sugar is ultimately converted into fat.

Atkins does not altogether ignore fats. He points out that trans fats are the dietary link to elevated cholesterol and heart disease. Trans fats lower the good HDL cholesterol and raise LDL (bad) cholesterol and lipoproteins. Trans fats also reduce responsiveness to insulin and block the uptake of essential fatty acids.

Atkins also emphasizes the selection of "safe food" products with the avoidance of most foods which contain antibiotics or hormones. He further advocates taking a wide variety of foods which will supply an array of vitanutrients and phytochemicals, and avoids any potential of addiction to a particular food stuff.

The first objective of the Atkins diet is to stabilize blood sugar. This is achieved by eliminating most simple carbohydrates and sugar containing foods and replacing them with either complex carbohydrates or non-carbohydrates (Table 28).

Table 28

Atkins Diet: Very low carbohydrate
Claims—Easy to stay with
—Age defying
—Boosts immunity
—Enhances brain function
—Reduces cardiovascular disease
—Combats diabetes

The diet is thus based on a much higher than normal fat and protein content. A second objective is to create a diet which is low in foods that create oxygen free radicals and high in the antioxidants that fight them. To increase antioxidant capacity the diet is very high in fresh vegetables and low-sugar fruits such as berries.

An advantage of the diet is that the patient does not have to count calories or even excessively restrict portion size. Steak and fish may be eaten with free access to fresh vegetables. Brown rice and genuine whole grain bread are allowed. Some cheeses are permitted without restriction but yogurts which are high in lactose, a simple sugar, should be kept to a minimum. Bran is allowed and nuts and seeds are permitted. Atkins recommends taking butter rather than margarine, stating that margarines contain large amounts of trans-fats, which release cascades of artery damaging free radicals. Fat intake also helps stabilize the blood sugar. Oils which are recommended are monounsaturated vegetable oils such as olive, almond, avocado, and macadamia. These oils are excellent sources of Omega-3 and Omega-6 essential fatty acids.

Replacement of simple carbohydrates with high-quality complex carbohydrates (starches) is advocated (Table 29). Complex carbohydrates are more likely to keep the blood sugar steady when they are combined with protein and fat. With regard to vegetables, if they are green then they can, by and large, be eaten freely. This means generous and varied portions of salad greens, broccoli, kale, brussel sprouts, and green beans are allowed.

Vegetables such as carrots, beets, peas and winter squash are higher in carbohydrates though they are also high in anti-oxidants. If potatoes are eaten it is better to take them with the skin. Fruits should only be taken in moderation. They are a good source of fiber, vitamins, minerals and other essential nutrients but they contain significant amounts of simple carbohydrates, and fruit juices should be avoided. Canned fruits have virtually no nutritional value and they are loaded with added sugar and should be avoided.

Table 29

Atkins Diet

Allows complex carbohydrates
Bans trans fats
Emphasizes safe food
High in antioxidants
Allows fresh vegetables and some fruits

Allows

All meats and fish
Butter and some margarines
Cheeses and milk
Oils and avocado
Green vegetables
Low-sugar fruits

Bans

All refined carbohydrates
Sugar
Sodas
Cakes
Cookies
Canned fruits

On the Atkins diet it is important to drink large amounts of fluid (Table 31). It is recommended that at least 8, eight-ounce glasses of fluid should be taken daily. It is better to use filtered water than tap water. Teas and decaffeinated coffee are allowed. Alcoholic beverages may be taken in moderation. Several studies have shown that having a glass of red wine has a beneficial effect on the heart and blood vessels. There is a lot of uncertainty relating to alcohol intake and it is wiser to drink either dry wine or straight liquor with a sugarless mixture such as a diet soda. Beer and dessert wines should be avoided (Table 30).

Table 30

Atkins Diet Drinks Allowed

8, eight-ounce glasses of water per day
Teas
Coffee—only decaffeinated
Diet sodas only
Red wine (no beers)

(Caffeine increases appetite and the rate of gastric emptying)

Convenience of Atkins

Difficult to overeat if you keep to the correct foods.
Without refined carbohydrates—satiety is produced earlier.
Ketones are produced.

Ketones

Headache
Fatigue
Bad breath
Constipation
They rarely build up to any significant degree.

Table 31

Drinks—Are Important

Sodas are packed with sugar
If you drink sodas, drink "diet" (0 calories)
Drink as much water as you can!!—8 or more glasses per day.
Most sodas contain 9—10 spoons of sugar and over 200 calories—Avoid these at all costs!

In regard to the amount of food taken, Atkins recommends eating until comfortable. Food which is free of carbohydrates satisfies the appetite more rapidly. Overeating becomes almost impossible. It is recommended to take a large high protein breakfast and three full meals a day. Relatively speaking, vegetables have considerably more antioxidant per carbohydrate gram than fruit and thus represent a much more valuable dietary choice.

Choices among the fruits are berries of any kind. Frozen berries frequently have added sugar. A cup of blueberries has about ten grams of carbohydrates, which is only forty calories. Avocados are an excellent source of monounsaturated fat. There has been much talk recently about the importance of carotenoids. It is claimed that the carotenoid lycopene may help to prevent cancer, particularly cancer of the prostate. This has now been added to many of the over-the-counter vitamin preparations. Sources of these are dark green leafy vegetables and orange-colored foods such as carrots. It is found in highest concentrations in tomatoes.

Without carbohydrates the body does not burn fat efficiently and produces compounds called ketones which accumulate in the blood. These sometimes cause nausea, headache, fatigue, bad breath and constipation. They can put a strain on the kidneys. Whether this diet increases the risk of heart disease, vascular disease and even cancer remains controversial but it must be said that no real evidence of this exists and that the diet is associated with reduced levels of serum cholesterol.

The Sugar Buster's Diet

The Sugar Buster's Diet emphasizes that sugar is toxic. It is stressed that overproduction of insulin causes the body to store excess sugar as fat. Insulin further inhibits the mobilization of previously stored fat, and insulin signals the liver to make cholesterol. The Sugar Buster's Diet prohibits carbohydrates that cause an intense insulin secretion, these are the refined sugars. Foods which must be eliminated from the diet are potatoes, corn, white rice, bread from refined flour, beets, carrots, granulated sugar, corn syrup, molasses, honey, sugar colas and beer. Red wine is allowed with the Sugar Buster's Diet. For those who consume alcoholic beverages, the one that is most beneficial is red wine. Populations in countries with a higher relative consumption of red wine to other spirits experience a lower incidence of cardiovascular disease. Alcohol, however, is high in calories. With the Sugar Buster's Diet, exercise is regarded as a definite plus.

Modulating insulin therefore is the key to the Sugar Buster's Diet. Successfully controlling insulin is stated to allow the patient to unlock improved performance through health and nutrition. To control insulin it is fundamental that the intake of sugar is controlled and that refined carbohydrates are cut down to a minimum. Avoiding refined carbohydrates results in lower average insulin levels in the blood throughout any given period. This has a markedly beneficial effect on reducing fat synthesis and storage as well as mitigating other adverse influences which insulin has on the cardiovascular system. As with the Atkins philosophy here also, it is emphasized that refined carbohydrates are very rapidly absorbed resulting in the secretion of large quantities of insulin which promote fat deposition. Unrefined carbohydrates however, require more digestive breakdown before absorption. This slower absorption modulates insulin secretion and results in less fat synthesis and storage and consequently less weight gain (Table 32).

Table 32

Sugar Buster's Diet—"Light the grill and throw away the frying pan."

Encourages lean meat:	Beef
	Fish
	Fowl
Also encourages:	Eggs
	Cheese
	Nuts

NO REFINED CARBOHYDRATES

The Sugar Buster's Diet thus does not ban all carbohydrates. There is particular emphasis on avoiding refined sugars. Many diets advocate eliminating almost all fat and meat, especially red meat. Although many people do eat too much fat, some fat in the diet is necessary to synthesize steroids, lipoproteins and other substances necessary for the proper metabolic operations of the body. Ingested fat plays little role in excessive fat accumulation in the body. Most of the excessive fat is due to the conversion of ingested carbohydrates to fat. Proponents of the Sugar Buster's diet place great emphasis on the eating of meat. Ingested protein stimulates glucagon secretion as well as providing the building blocks for the body. Glucagon promotes the breakdown of stored fat and helps counteract the effects of high insulin levels on the cardiovascular system.

Red Wine and Alcohol

In the Sugar Buster's Diet alcohol, in reasonable amounts, is considered beneficial. Alcohol increases HDL cholesterol and decreases platelet stickiness and aggregation which can lead to thrombosis. These actions tend to reduce the development of arteriosclerosis and are particularly likely to be achieved when red wine, rather than other forms of alcohol, is ingested. It has been shown in a number of studies that the number of deaths from cancer, heart disease, strokes and accidents are cumulatively reduced in people who take one or two alcoholic beverages per day but not more than three. Those who drink more than three run a higher relative risk of death from all causes (Table 33).

Table 33

Sugar Buster's Strategy

To modulate insulin production by withdrawing sugars with high glycemic indices.
Multiple small meals are preferable to one or two large ones.
Calories are not counted.
Drinking large amounts of water is encouraged.

The proponents of Sugar Busters place emphasis on eating patterns. Multiple meals stimulate less overall insulin secretion than one or two large feedings. Long periods of fasting alter the body's response to insulin by causing it to enter the conservation mode. This tends to increased fat storage. It is therefore recommended that we should strive to consume three balanced meals every day.

In the Atkins diet it is stated not to be necessary to count calories. It is also not necessary to count sugar grams, fat grams, or protein grams. Overall food intake is not restricted, provided that it consists of high-fiber carbohydrates, lean meats and unsaturated fats. Unlike the Atkins diet, Sugar Busters expresses concern about eating too much fat, especially saturated fats. With multiple meals per day, portion size is very important. The portions of food selected for each meal should fit on the bottom of the plate and should not extend over the sides, second and third helpings are discouraged. It is beneficial to consume calories early in the day and the eating of large meals late at night is forbidden. Ingested cholesterol, it is thought, leads to elevations in serum cholesterol and deposition of cholesterol in the arterial system. Between-meal snacks should consist of fruits with the exception of watermelons, pineapples, raisins and bananas which have a high glycemic index. Fruits contain the basic sugar fructose and stimulate approximately one-third of the insulin secretion which is created by glucose. Consequently, fruit alone as a snack is beneficial. Taken in combination with other carbohydrates it loses the advantage of lowering insulin secretion that is achieved when eaten by itself. Fruit should be eaten whole and fruit juices are discouraged. Sugar Busters recommend consuming fluids between, and particularly before, meals rather than at the time of eating. They discourage overconsumption of regular coffee and tea which can present a problem of too much caffeine. Caffeine makes the stomach secrete acid, which stimulates appetite.

Here also, as with the Atkins diet, it is advocated that a conscientious effort should be made to drink six or eight glasses of water per day. Drinking water throughout the day will lessen the desire for food thereby helping weight control. Breakfast cereals are discouraged. Most breakfast cereals are laced with either white sugar, brown sugar, molasses, corn syrup or honey. In fact it is difficult to purchase a pure, natural-grain cereal. The wheat bread which is allowed is whole grain, rather than whole meal (Table 34).

Table 34

Sugar Buster's Diet

Somewhat more liberal with carbohydrates than the
Atkins Diet.

Banned Carbs:
- Potatoes
- Corn
- White Rice
- White Bread
- Beets
- Carrots
- Sugar (granulated)
- Corn syrup
- Molasses
- Honey
- Sodas
- Beer

The Sugar Buster's Diet is aimed at reducing insulin secretion while enhancing the secretion of glucagon. This method of eating reduces body fat and cholesterol as well as many health problems caused by both of them. Dietary sources of protein are a must. Forms of lean meat, such as beef, fish and fowl are recommended. These should be grilled, baked or broiled since frying involves the use of saturated fats. Other excellent and healthy protein sources are eggs, cheese and nuts. They use the aphorism of "lighting the grill and throwing away the frying pan." Sugar Busters claim to be creating a new nutritional lifestyle. It is logical, practical and reasonable. It aims at removing unnecessary fat, especially saturated fat from the diet, and concentrating on the ingestion of lean and trimmed meats. Refined carbohydrates are strictly forbidden. Starches may be taken in moderation.

South Beach Diet

The South Beach Diet claims to be neither low carb nor low fat. The aim is to teach reliance on the right carbohydrates and the right fats—the good ones—and enable the patient to live quite happily without the bad carbs and bad fats. The claim is that between eight and thirteen pounds can be lost in the first two weeks. This is achieved by eating normal-size helpings of chicken, turkey, fish and shellfish. Plenty of vegetables are allowed and the diet includes eggs, cheese and nuts (Table 35). Salads are encouraged, using olive oil as a dressing. Three balanced meals a day are allowed and eating until hunger is satisfied is encouraged. Mid-morning and mid-afternoon snacks are permitted and dessert may be taken after dinner. Bread, rice, potatoes, pasta and baked goods are completely prohibited, as is fruit, in the early days (Table 36). Cakes, cookies, ice cream, and sugar are also banned in the early stages of the diet. Alcohol of any kind is ultimately allowed. In the early stages wine is permitted. It is claimed that most of the weight loss in the first two weeks comes off the abdomen so that clothes sizes already are influenced and physical cravings for food usually disappear for as long as the patient adheres to the program. It is claimed that patients are eating fewer of the foods that created those urges in the first place, and also fewer of the foods that caused the body to store excess fat. After the first two weeks, phase two is entered. Here fruit is allowed and a small amount of rice or cereal may be introduced. The subject continues on this phase until the ideal weight is achieved. Thereafter, in phase three, the subject is requested, permanently, to stay on a less restricted form of the diet and this will become a way of life.

Table 35

South Beach Diet

Allows: (Lean)

Beef
Pork
Veal
Lamb
Eggs
Chicken
Turkey
Fish

Nuts
Low-fat cheeses
Yogurt
Olive oil
Canola oil
Peanut oil

Table 36

South Beach Diet: The Right Carbohydrates and the Right Fats

Encourages:

Salads
Eggs
Cheese
Nuts
Olive oil

Bans:

Bread
Rice
Potato
Pasta
Cakes
Cookies
Ice Cream

It is of interest that the South Beach Diet was devised by Arthur Agatston, a cardiologist who had grown disillusioned with the low-fat, high-carbohydrate diet that the American Heart Association recommended. As a consequence he introduced the South Beach Diet in the mid 1990s. Focus was placed on the prevention of the myriad of heart and vascular problems that stemmed from obesity. While placing emphasis on beneficial effects to the cardiovascular system, Dr. Agatston also realizes the importance of the cosmetic effects of losing weight as a strong motivating factor for continuation with the diet. The physiological lift that comes from an improved appearance benefits the entire person and keeps many a patient from backsliding. The end result is cardiovascular health, with a better more active and more positive body habitus and attitude. The diet is also aimed at treating Syndrome X.

An important principle of the South Beach Diet is to permit good carbohydrates (fruits, vegetables, and whole grains) to be taken and curtail the bad carbohydrates (the highly processed ones—all of the fiber has been stripped away during manufacturing). To make up for the cut in carbohydrates, the diet permits ample fats and animal proteins. The reason for this is that the so-called "heart healthy" diets were very difficult to stick to, because they relied too heavily on the dieter's ability to eat low fat over the long-term. The South Beach Diet permits lean beef, pork, veal and lamb.

This diet also allows egg yolks which contain a lot of vitamin E and have a positive effect on the balance between good and bad cholesterol. Chicken, turkey, fish (especially the oily ones such salmon, tuna and mackerel) are recommended along with nuts, lowfat cheeses and yogurt. Olive oil, canola oil and peanut oil are allowed. These contain good fats. One of Agatston's criticisms of the Atkins diet is that the severe limitation of carbohydrates leads to the breakdown of fats, producing ketosis. To otherwise healthy overweight individuals, this is probably not harmful but may be associated with the decrease in blood volume and some dehydration which could affect kidney function and possibly, in the long term, cause permanent renal damage.

Another objection to Atkins diet, theoretically, is that following a meal of saturated fats there is dysfunction in the arteries which results in the lining of the inside of vessels with cholesterol plaques and thus the predisposition to thrombosis. These adverse effects do not occur when unsaturated fats are consumed.

In a randomized controlled clinical trial, including forty over-weight volunteers, the South Beach Diet was compared to the American Heart Association Program. After twelve weeks, five patients on the American Heart Association Diet had given up, compared to just one on the South Beach Plan. South Beach Dieters experienced a mean weight loss of 13.6 pounds, almost double the 7.5 pounds lost by the Heart Association group. Those on the South Beach Diet also showed a greater decrease in waist-to-hip ratio, suggesting a true decrease in cardiac risk. Cholesterol levels dramatically decreased for those on the South Beach Diet and their good-to-bad cholesterol ratio improved more than that of the Heart Association group. It is plain that much of the insulin resistance syndrome disappears after the initial two weeks on the South Beach Diet. The cravings for sugars and starches also, are virtually gone.

After two weeks, fruits and bran or oatmeal are allowed. At this stage a little whole-grain bread can also be introduced into the diet. It should not be spread with jelly but with butter. Potatoes are banned. Eggs should be boiled or poached and not fried. Fruits, which have the lowest glycemic index, are strawberries, blueberries and raspberries and are allowed. Bananas have a high glycemic index and should be avoided; tomato ketchup is not allowed as it is loaded with sugars. Tomato slices, however, are fine. Lettuce, pickles and onions are perfect. Green peppers, garlic, mushrooms, mustard and olives are good. Raw broccoli is excellent. Broccoli is covered with a layer of nutritious fiber and the carbohydrate content is slowly absorbed. Not only is the frying of potatoes bad, but even when boiled the glycemic index is high, as boiling makes the carbohydrate content more suitable for rapid absorption. The digestion of fats and proteins along with the carbohydrate, which is allowed, slows the speed with which the carbohydrates are rendered suitable for absorption.

A little olive oil will enhance this process of slowing down the absorption of the carbohydrate. Hence the practice, which is often recommended, of taking a spoonful of Metamucil in a glass of water about fifteen minutes before a meal. Non-soluble fiber mixed with the food has the effect of slowing the speed with which the stomach digests and also the rate at which the stomach empties is slowed, thus reducing the rate of absorption of carbohydrates.

Words of Warning—The Importance of What We Drink

In many ways what we drink is more critical than what we eat! The stomach empties liquids rapidly, rendering them suitable for quick absorption and therefore carbohydrate-containing liquids have an extremely high glycemic index. As has been pointed out, there is something of the order of nine or ten teaspoons of sugar in a can of Coke. If pure water is drunk, it has the effect of diluting the content of the stomach and slowing down the absorption of solid foods. Therefore water, at least eight glasses per day, is recommended.

Beer has a high glycemic index as a result of its maltose content, which makes it even worse than table sugar. Wine and whiskey are safer bets because they are made from different grains, vegetables or fruits. Red wine, in particular, is healthy with its proven cardiac benefits. Coffee is not necessarily bad, however the caffeine content does stimulate the stomach to secrete acid and thereby increases the rate of digestion, this has the same effect on gastric emptying, and it may increase appetite. Tea also contains caffeine and may be useful in the prevention of cardiac disease and possibly prostate cancer. According to the protagonist of the South Beach Diet, wine is less damaging than white bread—it's less fattening! (Table 37).

Table 37

Augmenting the South Beach Diet

(According to cardiologist Dr. Agatston.)
Aspirin.
Multivitamin preparations.
Fish oil—Omega 3 fatty acids.
Cholesterol-lowering drugs such as Lipitor or Zocor if indicated.
Testosterone gel!

The Glycemic Index

The glycemic index of a food is a measure of the amount the food increases your blood sugar compared, to the amount that the

90

same quantity of white bread would increase it. Low glycemic foods satisfy hunger longer and minimize food cravings better. With regard to bakery products, cakes and muffins tend to have a slightly lower glycemic index than bread but doughnuts and waffles have higher indexes (Table 38). Oats, bran, whole-meal bread and mixed grain bread have a lower glycemic index, but the glycemic index of gluten-free wheat bread and French baguettes is 30 percent higher. All bran, oatmeal and Special K have glycemic indexes of less than 80, whereas Rice Krispies and Corn Flakes are 50 percent higher than white bread. Barley, rye, and wheat, pure cereal grains, have glycemic indexes of 36 percent, 48 percent, and 59 percent respectively. Most dairy foods have relatively low glycemic indexes, that for lowfat yogurt, artificially sweetened, being only 20 percent; milk is 39 percent and fat-free milk is 46 percent. Ice cream has a glycemic index of 87 percent.

Glycemic indices of fruits vary from 32 percent, for cherries, to 103 percent for watermelons. Grapefruit, peaches, oranges and pears have a glycemic index of less than 50 percent. Bananas and pineapples are much higher, 89 percent and 94 percent, respectively. Legumes have indices ranging from soy beans at 23 percent to canned baked beans at 70 percent. Vegetables range from sweet potatoes at 63 percent, carrots at 70 percent, mashed potato at 100 percent, fries at 107 percent, to baked potatoes at 158 percent. With regard to sugars themselves, the glycemic index of glucose is 137 percent, of maltose, found in beer, 150 percent, lactose 92 percent but that of fructose is only 32 percent.

The following vegetables have a glycemic index of less than 20 percent; artichoke, asparagus, broccoli, brussel sprouts, cabbage, cauliflower, celery, cucumbers, beets, kale, mustard greens, spinach, turnips, mushrooms, nuts, peppers and green beans (Tables 43–48).

Table 38

The Glycemic Index of Food

The amount that the food in question increases your blood sugar compared with the amount that the same weight of white bread would increase it.
Avoid white bread—Glycemic index = 100

Effects of Glycemic Indices

High glycemic index foods continue to stimulate your appetite. Low glycemic index foods minimize food cravings.

Table 39

Glycemic Indices Greater than 1.0

Doughnuts
Waffles
Gluten-free bread
French baguettes
Bagels
Watermelons!
Mashed potato
French fries
Baked potato: 158 percent

Table 40

Foods with Glycemic Indices Less than 20 Percent

Artichoke
Asparagus
Broccoli
Brussel sprouts
Cabbage
Cauliflower
Celery
Cucumbers
Beets
Kale
Mustard greens
Spinach
Turnips
Mushrooms
Nuts (but high fat content)
Peppers
Green beans

Table 41

Glycemic Index of Sugars

Glucose	—	137 percent
Maltose	—	150 percent
Lactose	—	92 percent
Fructose	—	32 percent

Complex carbohydrates all have lower indices.

Table 42

Alcohol and the Glycemic Index

Best	Worst
Red wine—cardiac benefits	Beer (Maltose)
Whiskey	

Two glasses per day is beneficial—over that the situation deteriorates!

Table 43

Glycemic Index in Fruits

GOOD	BAD
Strawberries	Bananas
Blueberries	
Raspberries	
Red-Black	

Table 44

Glycemic Index in Vegetables: South Beach Diet

GOOD	BAD
Tomatoes	Potatoes
Lettuce	
Onions	
Pickles	
Green peppers	
Garlic	
Mustard greens	
Olives	
Broccoli	

Results of the South Beach Diet

It is common for people to lose eight to twelve pounds. in weight during the first two weeks of the South Beach Diet. This is very encouraging for diet participants, but most of the initial weight loss is due to reduced carbohydrate intake, which results in loss of water storage and water loss from restricting carbohydrate equalizes after about ten to fourteen days. Thereafter weight loss slows.

Proponents of the South Beach Diet strongly recommend an exercise program, but in moderation, so that the exercise program becomes only a slight intervention in normal lifestyle rather than a major new discipline. For most people a brisk twenty-minute daily walk is recommended but can only be expected to burn about 100 calories. The majority of benefit from exercise is gained during the first twenty minutes. Weight training has many benefits. It improves muscle-to-fat ratio, increases metabolism and promotes the body to burn fuel faster, even when sleeping. Increasing lean body mass, that is body weight from anything other than fat, is a helpful effect of weight lifting. Training is also helpful for women in preventing osteoporosis. Furthermore, exercise lowers blood pressure and increases good cholesterol. The developer of the South Beach Diet, Agatston, who is a cardiologist, in addition to adhering to his own diet from the point of view of preventing cardiac problems without necessarily promoting further weight loss, takes aspirin, fish oil capsules, and uses testosterone gel.

The Ornish Diet

The Ornish Diet is a high fiber, lowfat diet. The rationale is that fiber takes up a lot of room in the stomach, gives rise to early satiety and is ultimately poorly absorbed. Therefore in combination with a lowfat diet weight loss occurs. This diet keeps fat to no more than 10 percent of daily caloric intake and it is claimed that heart disease can be reversed. The diet is difficult to adhere to and produces only short-term satiety. This diet, like the preceeding low-carbohydrate diets, has been heavily promoted (Table 45).

Table 45

The Ornish Diet

Low fat—high fiber	
Fiber	Expands in the stomach
	Slows down food absorption
Fat	Less than 10 percent of daily caloric intake —possibly reverses arteriosclerosis and coronary artery disease

A much publicized diet.

Protein Power—The Eades Diet

This is essentially a low-carbohydrate diet and depends on the rationale that eating protein adds to lean body mass but does not stimulate insulin and therefore the overall effect is a slimmer and healthier body. Little emphasis is placed on reducing fat intake (Table 46).

Table 46

Other Disciplines

Protein Power—The Eades Diet.
Low carbohydrate—Low fat—High protein.
Natural hygiene.
Uses large amounts of water and aperients.
High water content vegetables contain fiber, vitamins and minerals.

Importance of Water in Diets

It must be said that most diets ultimately fail. That is largely because people tend to gradually stray away from the diet and ultimately, while becoming disillusioned, return to their old bad habits. It is suggested that one reason why diets fail is that they create too much personal thought about what the subject is going to eat—and this tends to stimulate appetite.

Another reason for failure is that people temporize on diets thinking that a six-week crash diet will produce the desired effect which even, if they managed to achieve it, is soon lost when the short period of dieting is over. It is safe to say that so much emphasis has been placed on diets and new diets through the media, television and magazines that if any of these were successful in the long term we would not now be facing such a massive increase in the number of obese people in the population.

All of the diets I have described place emphasis on drinking large amounts of water. At least eight glasses per day. A weight loss program that is now twenty years old depends not so much on diet as on what is described as "natural hygiene." The basic foundation of "natural hygiene" was that the body is always striving for health, which is achieved by continually cleansing itself of deleterious waste material. It is not achieved by drinking water alone, according to the proponents of natural hygiene, high-water-content foods are the key. These are essentially fruits and vegetables. It is argued that fruits and vegetables not only contain large amounts of water, but basically all of the essential vitamins and minerals required for good health.

It has long been known that there are certain groups of people in the world who live extraordinary long periods of time while maintaining good health. These long lived people are the Abkhazians of Russia, the Vilcabanbans of Ecuador and the Hunzukuts of Pakistan. There is no obesity in these societies and they live amazingly disease-free lives. It is also claimed that there is neither cancer nor heart disease. Their diet is essentially comprised of fruits and vegetables.

XIV
Supermarkets—The Food We Buy

It is important to be careful about the consumption of foods bought from supermarkets. For example, more fat is found in three slices of bread than in a calorie-rich Mars bar. Some breakfast cereals contain more than 15 percent fat and some best-selling ready-made meals have more than triple the fat of other similar products. The amount of fat in pizzas can vary from fifteen to four percent. Supermarkets provide often unchallenging comfort cuisine, rows and rows of ready-made foods from chicken pot pies to sponge cakes that once would have been made at home. These products contain palm oil emulsifiers, hydrogenated vegetable oil and a bewildering array of additives. These are used partly to ensure that foods last longer, taste better and cost less. Fat is abundant, cheap and can prolong the shelf life of products, adding an attractive texture. The result, over the past few decades, has been rising fat contents in many of the most popular foods.

Product longevity is an issue here. For example, a homemade lemon cake containing 10 percent fat would be stale and inedible after two or three days, while a supermarket cake with 20 percent fat tastes the same in three months as it does now. Fat emulsifiers are based on the chemistry which came out of the soap industry. They make fat more palatable. The result is that some breads contain 12 percent fat whereas, in contrast, full-fat milk contains only 4 percent fat. According to the Atkins philosophy, this might not seem to be so important, but in all probability it is and possibly extremely so. The reason being that trans-fatty acids from hydrogenated vegetable fat used in cakes, cookies and margarine are in themselves a health risk. Trans-fatty acids cannot properly be digested and the body simply stores them. There is evidence that trans-fatty acids are involved in the formation of cholesterol deposits in blood vessels in diabetes and in obesity. On the other hand, monounsaturated fats such as those found in avocados and nuts are believed to be beneficial in moderation, possibly protecting against heart disease.

It may be, therefore, that all of the obesity revolution is not the responsibility of the consumer, but is contributed to, to some significant extent, by supermarkets which control about 90 percent of food consumption. Supermarkets are presently going some way to provide healthy alternatives and labeling of energy content in food is increasingly being practiced. In the United Kingdom, a House of Commons Select Committee has recently criticized the food industry for not doing enough to promote healthy foods. They are introducing a traffic-light system policy for labeling foods, those with increasing caloric intake, being in the red zone.

A study reported in July, 2004, involved 126 nutrition professionals with the American Dietetic Association, including sport nutritionists, cookbook and nutrition book authors, heads of hospital wellness programs, university weight loss researchers and many dieticians in private practice. These national obesity researchers agreed that we cannot afford to allow the overweight population to increase over the next twenty years as it has over the last equivalent period. It was emphasized that a strategy must be formulated to prevent the 1 to 2 pounds that the average American gains each year. About 65 percent of adults in the U.S.A. now weigh too much. This study determined the following major obstacles: 1) Most people do not have a realistic idea of portion sizes. Restaurants often contribute to the problem with portions that are at least twice the recommended serving size; 2) Children don't change bad eating habits for good; instead they choose fad diets which they adhere to in the short term only and then revert to their previous eating habits; 3) Most people consider exercise a drudgery and rarely stay with exercise programs; 4) There is a large reluctance to change eating habits as people become "addicted" to their favorite foods; 5) People fail to realize that there is no such thing as a miracle diet. What the overweight want to hear is that losing weight is quick, easy, miraculous and involves little effort. No such system exists. The nutritionists in this study felt that a big problem was that activity had been squeezed out of people's lives by modern technology. Moving from cars, to desks, to television screens and computers, has ruled exercise out of most people's way of existence.

XV

Visiting the Supermarket—What to Purchase

Wherever we go today we are faced with a plethora of multiple food items which are on sale. Even at the gas station, quite a large array of foods are available, chiefly fast foods and those which are high in carbohydrate and fat content. These are also relatively inexpensive. Clearly, buying and taking into the house the wrong type of food is a fundamental problem in the obesity equation and if bad food is not available in the house, then it is not going to be eaten during periods of vulnerability. It is important, therefore, in carrying out grocery shopping that healthy foods are purchased and those which are harmful to health or have a particularly high glycemic index should be avoided.

When visiting the supermarket, go easy on breads, rice, cereals and pasta. There is no need to eat breakfast cereals and very little need to eat bread. Pasta is also something which can readily be avoided. When bread is purchased it should be the whole-meal or whole-wheat variety and white sliced bread should be avoided. Pizzas should be avoided as should cakes, bagels, and cookies. There is no need to have refined granulated sugar in the house. When entering the supermarket you are usually faced with an array of the foregoing foodstuffs. Resist the temptation to buy them and move on to the fruits and vegetables section.

Here, not only are the glycemic indexes lower and the number of calories taken less, but also these foods contain essential vitamins and minerals which are important for health. When in this section go for green-colored items such as lettuce, broccoli, asparagus and spinach. Vegetables are better than fruits and fruits which are somewhat undesirable are bananas and melons. The only fruits and vegetables which contain a significant amount of fat is avocado, but this is healthy fat and good eating. There is also some fat in coconuts. Ultimate time-saving purchases can be prepared salads which are readily available and do not involve any cooking. Roots which are dark red, purple or black are often healthy eating but jams and jellies like blueberry jellies often have a considerable amount of added sugar.

Along the dairy aisle, lowfat dairy products are an excellent source of food and nutrition and contain important minerals such as calcium which are essential, particularly in women, to prevent metabolic bone disease. Buy either skim or 1 percent lowfat milk. Fat-free milk may be fortified with additional protein and along with that contains more calcium. Lowfat cottage cheese, sour cream and yogurt are healthy foods and lowfat cheese is a good addition to the diet. One of the best cheeses along these lines is mozzarella. Solid dressings like ranch should be avoided, but honey mustard need not contain too much sugar and buttermilk garlic on the whole contains little fat. Eggs are a useful source of protein and despite the cholesterol content of the yolk are not a bad form of nutrition.

When entering the meat area, concentrate on lean white meat. Turkey and chicken slices can contain less than 4 percent fat or even no fat at all. Steak, in particular sirloin and tenderloin can be eaten once or twice a week but the fat should be removed. Even pork is healthy eating provided the fat is taken off. In the poultry section, white poultry is lower in fat than dark. The skin of turkeys, chickens and duck is high in fat and calories and should be removed. Seafood is excellent, particularly white fish. Great emphasis has been placed on eating salmon, which always had a great reputation. This has, however, been somewhat tarnished by adverse publicity relating to carcinogens which are present in farm-raised salmon. There is some dispute about the authenticity of these claims and although the carcinogens probably exist, they are most likely present only in minute quantities and thus unlikely to affect health adversely.

Tofu is an excellent source of both protein and calcium. Nuts can be bought because they are possibly helpful in preventing cardiovascular disease. You will need to buy some butter or margarine and it probably does not matter which, provided that the margarine does not contain too many trans-fatty acids. Purchase low- or no-calorie sweeteners such as Splenda. Adverse publicity about saccharin, which is high in Sweet-n-lo, causing various forms of cancer probably represents an exaggeration. Almost everyone tolerates sweeteners well. Some react adversely to the aspartane content of some sweeteners such as Equal. Whatever the downside of eating sweeteners these are very much less than those associated with ingesting large amounts of sugar.

It is important therefore when visiting the supermarket to employ the right strategy because what you walk out with is certainly what you are going to eat and probably gives as good a reflection as anything of the way in which your food intakes relate to your health and weight.

XVI

Behavioral Therapy

Behavioral techniques are often based on close monitoring and peer pressure. They frequently involve keeping a record of all food and drink consumed and of all physical activities. Programs are often individually tailored to suit personality and lifestyle. Self-help groups frequently play an important role in this form of therapy and often mentors are available at any time to help when the patient is experiencing difficulty.

The detailed documentation of the patient's eating habits and exercise forms an important base of self-education and this can then be manipulated appropriately. Once the principal elements underlying the subject's behavior have been established, certain disciplines are invoked. The patient is advised to sit down to all meals, adhere to a fixed-time controlled eating regime, eat slowly, avoid snacks and drink plenty of water. They are advised to resist the temptation to purchase inappropriate food items for the home. Weighing of these subjects takes place about once every two weeks. Peer group meetings are frequently held. Peer pressure is an important stimulus to the patient to adhere to the program. The most widely known system which adheres to this sort of philosophy is Weight Watchers.

Boredom and inactivity are common reasons for eating. Those who are engaged in stimulating and creative mental activity are much less likely to snack while working. If, however, calories are restricted to too great an extent then the subject becomes increasingly focused on eating. The way around this is to eat celery, drink water or stop working and take frequent walks. Some individuals eat excessively when under stress. It has been shown that obese women are more emotionally reactive and more likely to engage in emotional eating than women of normal weight. The more emotional the women are feeling, the more likely they are to eat.

A common feature noticed among obese people is that when in company they eat either the same amount as others or even sometimes markedly less. In contrast, when alone, they tend to binge eat. Behavioral therapy focuses on dealing with the emotional factors which effect eating.

Other ways of overcoming an intense desire to eat are by making a phone call to friends so as to relieve loneliness and anxiety or by sending an e-mail to someone who has a similar problem. Obesity leads to social isolation and that in itself is a stimulus to eating for many people. Being dissatisfied with one's own weight is in itself a factor which predisposes to the above kind of conditions and can be a stimulus to eating. Surveys of women have shown that while most women are self-conscious about some aspect of their appearance, most focus their attention on their weight and over eighty percent of women claim that they would like to be slimmer. This situation has been accentuated by the modern tendency to choose extremely thin women as fashion models. These extremely thin women are often those bordering on anorexia. The ideal shape of a woman as manifest by art and advertising can be illustrated by the change which has occurred from the time of Rubens and Rembrandt, where women were voluptuous, to the 1950s where the ideal was portrayed by Marilyn Monroe, to the present day where the Calvin Klein underwear advertisements reveal only skin and bone! The same to some extent is true for men, where models are usually tall and thin. Society dictates how people should look and in reality, achieving these ideals is difficult or impossible for most. The inability to achieve them may be associated with failure, giving rise to people either opting out of the race or, as a result of the anxiety which it produces, overeating as a rebound phenomenon.

Controlled clinical trials of behavioral therapy have shown that patients lose about ten pounds in the first eight to ten weeks. During that time, compliance tends to be good and dropout rates are low. With increasing periods of time, however, many members abandon the program and maintenance of weight loss beyond one year is rare. A large study of behavioral therapy programs showed that 16 percent maintained their weight loss of over forty pounds and 17 percent were heavier than at the start of the program. People investing in behavioral treatments therefore can expect to achieve results as good as, if not better than, those which are achieved by drug therapy. The results of both of these treatment modalities, in the long term, however, are very disappointing. No one has adequately assessed the problem of long-term maintenance. Systems of rewards have been used and these appear only to be valuable in the short term. Similarly, the use of penalties appears to be ineffective over time. Perhaps the most important adjunct to this form of therapy is social support and with close interdependence, results tend to be better. Enthusiasts can now communicate instantly by e-mail in the hope of gaining help and overcoming the tendency to depart from the strict constraints of the program. Studies have shown that individual treatment by a therapist produces better results than group therapy.

Although behavioral therapy is designed to provide a set of skills to identify and modify inappropriate eating, to stimulate exercise and good thinking habits, these programs most frequently, ultimately end in failure and weight is regained.

Another form of therapy which could broadly be included under the heading of behavioral is psychiatric management. Society is geared to the ingestion of calorie-dense food, there has been portion-size inflation and foods of high fat and carbohydrate content are the most heavily advertised products on television. Furthermore, obesity leads to depression and depression is commonly associated with binge eating or eating to achieve solace. Psychiatric management combines with cognitive therapy. An eating laboratory may be used to instruct the patients in the basics of nutrition. Drugs are frequently used as an adjunct. Psychotherapy plays a role and support contact through e-mail also is advocated.

Individuals are motivated by different factors. One patient, who lost 130 pounds, did so because she became frustrated on a hike with her teenage daughter. The woman was so winded after walking a short distance that she had to sit down on a bench. An elderly man with a cane passed her by, as did a person in a wheelchair. This was the straw that broke the camel's back. It was that image that she kept in her mind every time she was tempted with things like a plate of cookies or some high-calorie food. She would repeat to herself, "If this is going to stop my chances of hiking with my daughter, it's not worth it."

Other patients are similarly motivated by discovering that they are unable to get into the clothes they wish to buy. Similarly, they see that those clothes which do fit them are either hard to obtain or singularly unattractive. Conversely, some are loath to go on diets because they feel they will never be able to eat their favorite foods again. This is far from the truth. Specially designed diets exist which can incorporate favorite foods without resulting in excess caloric intake. A good rule of thumb is the eighty-twenty rule. About 80 percent of foods eaten should be lean protein, such as poultry, fish and beans, fruits and vegetables, lowfat dairy such as yogurt and skim milk, high-fiber grain products and healthier fat such as olive oil. The other 20 percent of the time they can eat foods that are not so healthful. No one is saying weight loss is easy, it takes a lot of work and may be expensive. It is hard to change lifelong habits and to purchase different foods which have to be fixed in different ways and which are sometimes more expensive than those previously bought. It is financially viable in the long term, by reducing the obesity associated morbidity that will inevitably ultimately accrue.

XVII

Behavioral Therapy—Should You Join a Group?

Behavioral therapy programs depend upon the effects of peer pressure. They offer differing disciplines underlying the strategy for weight loss but all involve group meetings, where participants compare results and share problems. The atmosphere is one which creates commitment and applies pressure in order for the patient to achieve results. Patients can often choose the approach that suits them best. Approaches often depend upon calorie counting but "no-counting plans" also exist. Programs vary in terms of group size and number of visits required. Some of these programs not only spell out exact data requirements but require the purchase of special meals. A number of these plans exist online and others involve Internet weight loss companionship for Weight Watchers meetings. These provide access to recipes and tools to those who are already attending meetings, allegedly making it easier to stay on the plan and see progress.

Weight Watchers is the largest of these plans and provides individualized diets which are based on a point system. There is flexibility in choice of foods and it is possible to earn extra points by exercising but it is essential that the allocated number of points is not exceeded. The Weight Watchers Flex Plan allows subjects to enjoy the full range of food options while making better choices within the point system. Any food can be chosen. The essential factor is being in control of how much is eaten. An alternative to the Flex Plan is the Core Plan which focuses on wholesome foods without calorie counting. Patients are allowed to eat from a list of wholesome foods from all food groups. It is stated that they can enjoy satisfying eating without "empty calories" and they are allowed an occasional treat in controlled amounts.

Weight Watchers meetings provide coaching and insights in order to help the subject reach their goal. They are taught to make wise choices, eat healthily, and enjoy a combination of food and exercise. The support and guidance are major factors in enabling them to reach their goal and stay there. Participants in the plan benefit from the practical experiences, tips and peer pressure of others losing weight with Weight Watchers. Along with the meeting, Weight Watchers online provides interactive resources, encouraging following of the plan in a step-by-step way online. Access tips and strategies are provided to encourage following of the plan. It is stated that this makes it easy to manage food choices and activities and discover many delicious recipes. In addition, the Internet weight-loss companion gives e-mail addresses for subjects to contact peers in times of need.

Weight Watchers staff include registered dieticians, exercise physiologists and clinical psychologists. Lifetime members may become leaders who deliver the program to participants. The average cost of Weight Watchers is a one-time registration fee of $20.00 with a weekly fee of $10–$15. If the subject is qualified for lifetime membership then it is free. Some twenty-thousand meetings are held weekly within North America. Patients are encouraged to attend meetings once per week for about one hour. There is no formal contract so fees are only paid for meetings attended. Each week there is a confidential weigh-in to measure progress. Advice is given on making wise choices, eating healthily and enjoying food and exercise. Every week new tips and program materials are given.

The Weight Watchers program leader explains the strategy and identifies goals. Meeting leaders are usually people who have had successful outcomes from the Weight Watchers program. They undergo formal training in the plan and are committed to the success and to their own maintenance of weight loss. Subjects also benefit from tips, recipes and others' experiences. Members can sign up for Weight Watchers E-tools and online weight loss advice. Getting started is easy once the patient provides their zip code, local meetings are identified online and the atmosphere is altogether friendly and positive. With the Flex Plan, subjects are given a point calculator and points tracker, a list of over a thousand recipes and points value for these recipes. A Flex Plan restaurant guide is even given to provide advice when eating out. Access is available around the clock. For the Core Plan the patient is given a comprehensive core food list with all of the essential foods they can enjoy without tracking or counting. They can browse hundreds of core recipes and core meal item ideas. Success is charted on a weight tracker and progress chart and a Core Plan restaurant guide exists.

The Jenny Craig program employs a philosophy based on exercise, lifestyle modification and the taking of a low calorie diet. Subjects are encouraged to eat three meals a day and three snacks. Much emphasis is placed on increased physical activity. Packaged foods are available and recommended particularly during the early phases. Weight loss of about one to two pounds per week is usually achieved which is similar to that on Weight Watchers. The staff involved in the Jenny Craig program are registered dieticians who work with trained non-medical personnel. The latter have completed a training session and participate in regular updating educational sessions. The Jenny Craig program is more expensive than Weight Watchers.

Opti-fast is a medically supervised rapid weight loss program which is administered in hospitals and clinics. The plan requires liquid meal replacements and food bars. Dietary requirements are stringent and participants are assigned to an 800, 950, or 1200 calorie package. This program is intended for those who are at least fifty pounds overweight and the program runs for approximately three months followed by a six week transitional period. Emphasis is placed on increased physical activity and individual counseling is available.

These programs are more expensive, often costing about three thousand dollars for the whole program. Health management resources provide medically supervised rapid weight loss programs for patients who are fifty pounds or more overweight. Diets as low as 500 calories per day are provided and these are monitored by medical personnel. Meal replacements and special foods need to be purchased in order to adhere accurately with the requirements of this program. Weekly meetings are held and weight loss of between one and five pounds a week is expected and frequently achieved. The programs are run by physicians, registered dieticians, nurses and psychologists. The cost of this program is about seventy dollars per week.

Some programs exist which place emphasis upon peer support but do not require a planned dietary structure. Structure of the staff supervising these programs is based on the provision of psychologists and registered dieticians. Psychologists place emphasis on developing internal skills of self-nurturing and adhering to limits to achieve a diet which is free from excess. Telecoaching is available through video conferencing centers.

All of these programs work to some extent, particularly in the early stages, though program abandonment is common and rebound weight gain can result. Most of these programs include physical activity recommendations and emphasis is placed on the importance of adhering to these. Once again there tends to be considerable fall off in adherence to programs of increased physical activity. Radical programs such as those which employ a diet of less than 1000 calories may be associated with certain health risks like an increased incidence of gallstones and their complications or even coronary artery disease. Cost is often an important factor in determining whether or not subjects participate in these programs. The least expensive of these programs is Weight Watchers.

XVIII

Appetite Suppressant Drugs in the Management of Obese Patients

Over the years, many appetite suppressants have been used, especially Fenfluramine, Phenteramine, and Mazindol and all these have been shown to lessen hunger and decrease food intake in normal weight subjects (Tables 47, 48). Fenfluramine has recently been withdrawn by the FDA as a result of its tendency to cause pulmonary hypertension, or lung damage, which occurs in a small number of individuals treated with this drug. These drugs are stimulants and tend to increase metabolic rate but their major role seems to be in appetite suppression.

Table 47

Categories of Drugs Used in the Treatment of Obesity

Sympathomimetics—Stimulants—Anorexiants
Dextroamphetamine (Addesall, Dexedrine)
Methylphenindate (Ritalin, Methylin Concerta)
Phenteramine (Adipex-P, Ionamin, Phentiride, Phentrercot, Teramine)
Sibutramine (Meridia)
Antidepressants
    Fluoxetine (Prozac)
    Sertraline (Zoloft)
    Imipramine (Tofranil)
    Buproprion (Wellbutrin)
(Not all antidepressants are effective. Some, such as Remeron, stimulate appetite and cause weight gain.)
Anticonvulsants
    Topiramate (Topamax)

Oral Hypoglycemic Agents
    Metformin
Herbal Products
    St. John's Wort
Fat absorption blockers
    Orlistat

Table 48

Drugs Used in the Treatment of Obesity

Phenteramine (Adipex-P, Ionamin, Phentiride, Phentrercot, Tera-
    mine, Profast, OBY-trim)
Sibutramine (Meridia)
Dextroamphetamine (Addesall, Dexedrine, Dextrastat)
Caffeine
Fluoxetine
Prozac
Zoloft
Wellbutrin
Topamax
Metformin

The majority of placebo-controlled double-blind clinical trials of appetite suppressant drugs in the management of obesity have shown a significantly greater loss of weight in those patients receiving the active drug. The effect is most noticeable in the first four weeks of treatment and thereafter weight loss decreases. Few trials have demonstrated continuing weight loss after periods of three to six months. Furthermore, after stopping drug therapy, a large proportion of weight is regained. Sometimes more is gained than has been lost. There is also a risk of drug dependency and drug abuse with these agents which are frequently related to the amphetamines. However, total dependence is unusual and the majority of obese patients find little difficulty in stopping these drugs.

Use of appetite suppressant drugs should, on the whole, be limited to those in whom there is a substantial risk to physical or mental health as a result of the obese state. Drugs may act as an adjunct to dieting or behavioral therapy. A combination of these modalities is frequently, in the short term, beneficial. The sudden withdrawal of these drugs can sometimes lead to overt depressive symptoms. Most weight-reducing drugs stimulate the sympathetic nervous system and therefore side effects include insomnia, restlessness, irritability, dry mouth and tachycardia, or rapid heart beat. They should not be used in patients with angina. Commonly reported adverse effects include nausea and diarrhea.

The first drug which was widely used in the treatment of obesity was phenteramine, which was introduced in the late 1950s. In the 1970s phenfluramine also became available and these two drugs were widely used in combination under the name fen-phen. In the late 1990s it became apparent that these drugs could be associated with cardiorespiratory problems and in consequence the drugs were withdrawn from the market. Prior to their withdrawal some fourteen million subscriptions were written for these drugs each year (Table 49).

Table 49

Side Effects of Weight-Reducing Drugs

Insomnia
Restlessness
Irritability
Dry mouth
Constipation
Tachycardia
Angina
Nausea
Vomiting
Diarrhea

Sibutramine (Meridia) is an appetite suppressant said to give a sensation of early satiety. Studies have shown a weight loss of about 10 percent of the starting weight at the end of one year. The drug is a stimulant and can increase blood pressure and cardiac rate thus significant concerns exist as to its use, particularly in the elderly.

Other drugs which are used as appetite suppressants are Tenuate Dospan, Didrex, Bontirl and Apidex. None of these agents are FDA approved for use in the treatment of obesity and the results of their use are unimpressive. The anti-depressants, Prozac, Zoloft, and Wellbutrin have been widely used in weight loss programs though they do not have an established role. Topamax is a drug which has been used with some success. It is fundamentally an anti-convulsant but also works as an appetite suppressant, sometimes it has produced impressive weight loss. Metformin, a drug used in diabetes, is thought to promote the more efficient use of glucose and may be effective in producing a small amount of weight loss, particularly in the Type II diabetic. An anti-depressant, which is available over the counter as a neutraceutical, is St. John's Wort. This drug seems to work like an S.S.R.I. type of anti-depressant.

A drug which has a totally different mode of action is Orlistat which blocks the absorption of fat from the intestinal tract. In a large study carried out by the European Obesity Study Group in the year 2000, Orlistat, which had been administered for two years, was shown to promote weight loss, minimize weight regain and improve lipid profile, blood pressure and quality of life. Diarrhea from the malabsorption of fat is a side effect of the use of this drug. The pharmaceutical companies, being well aware of the great potential which exists for an efficacious form of drug therapy, are currently carrying out a number of clinical trials on new agents but none of these has yet passed the FDA for routine use in the United States.

An experimental drug, Rimonabant, has shown considerable promise by disrupting the function of centers in the base of the brain. This drug is still at an early stage in terms of clinical trial data. Other potential areas for development include studies related to neuropeptide-Y and C75.

Much publicity has recently been associated with the use of Hoodia. This is an extract of a cactus plant exclusive to the Kalahari Desert in Southern Africa. The agent has been associated with the production of quite impressive amounts of weight loss though the mechanism of action is unknown.

Few patients treated with drugs reach their goal weight and almost none reach their ideal weight. Currently available drugs help to produce a mean weight loss of about 10 percent of body weight at the start of treatment. As obesity is a chronic, usually lifelong condition, the value of drugs is very limited and no "best drug" has really emerged. It is possible that combination therapy may be indicated. Not a single well-conducted study shows efficacy and safety of drug therapy in the long term.

XIX

Basic Anatomy of the Upper Gastro-Intestinal Tract

In order to understand the basics of the operations performed for obesity some knowledge of basic anatomy is necessary.

Esophagus

The esophagus or gullet is a muscular tube, ten inches in length, which runs from the back of the throat to the abdominal cavity. It passes vertically through the chest or thorax, behind the heart, and alongside the spine. The esophagus enters the abdomen by passing through the diaphragm and ends at the upper end of the stomach.

The esophagus is responsible for propelling food stuffs from the back of the throat into the upper stomach. This it does by a series of quite forceful contractions known as peristaltic waves. At its upper and lower ends are sphincters or valves. The valve at the lower end is responsible for preventing the reflux of stomach contents into the esophagus, a condition known as gastrointestinal reflux disease or GERD.

The Stomach

The stomach is a large muscular organ which acts as a reservoir for the storage of food which is passed into it from the esophagus. The stomach is "j" shaped and has a capacity of about 1.5 liters, but under normal resting conditions, when the stomach is empty, its volume is about fifty ccs. The stomach is a strong muscular organ. The musculature is responsible for the grinding of food stuffs and the converting of solid material, which has been swallowed, into a liquefied form, prior to releasing it lower down into the intestinal tract. The lining of the upper stomach secretes acid which starts to break down the ingested food stuffs and initiates the digestive process. At the lower end of the stomach is a thick muscular ring called the pylorus. This releases food stuffs from the stomach into the intestine in a highly coordinated manner. If the pylorus is damaged or bypassed, food stuffs can empty too rapidly and produce the symptoms of dumping (Figure 5).

The Duodenum

The duodenum is a "c" shaped tube of intestine, ten inches in length which connects the outlet of the stomach to the small intestine. Halfway along the duodenum, bile from the liver and juice from the pancreas enter it to mix with food stuffs. It is here that the major process of digestion is initiated.

The Pancreas

The pancreas is large organ which is stretched across the back of the abdomen and has two main functions. The first of these is the secretion of a fluid rich in bicarbonate which contains enzymes that are responsible for the major breakdown process of proteins, carbohydrates and fats. Its second function is a hormonal one, the secretion of the hormones insulin and glucagon which, as has been pointed out, is so intimately involved with the obesity process (Figure 6).

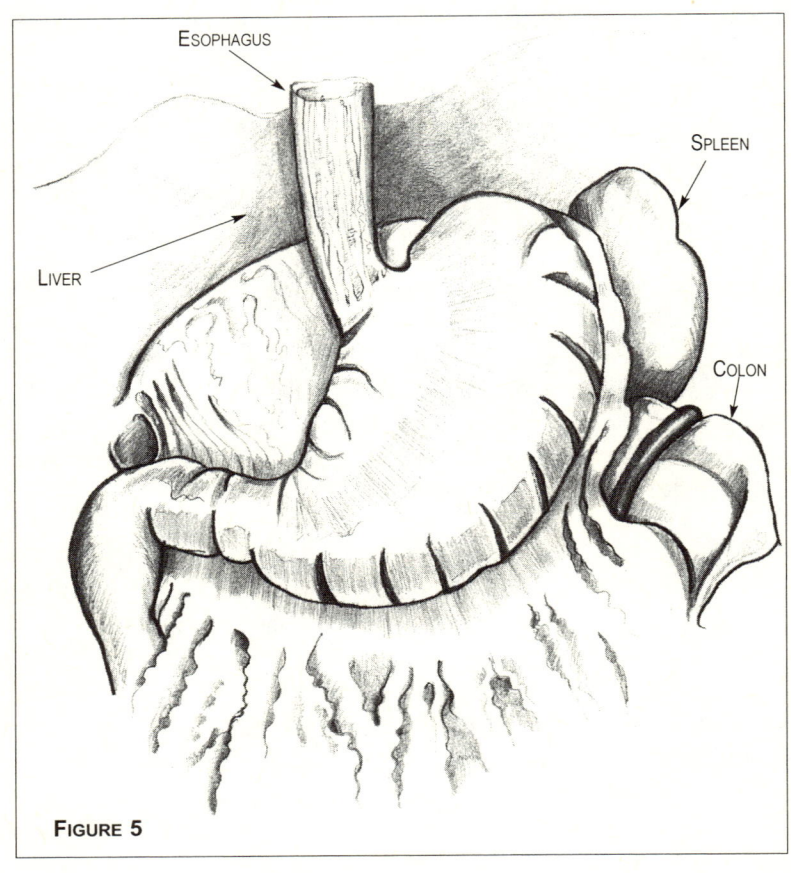

ESOPHAGUS

SPLEEN

LIVER

COLON

FIGURE 5

Anatomy of the gastrointestinal tract

118

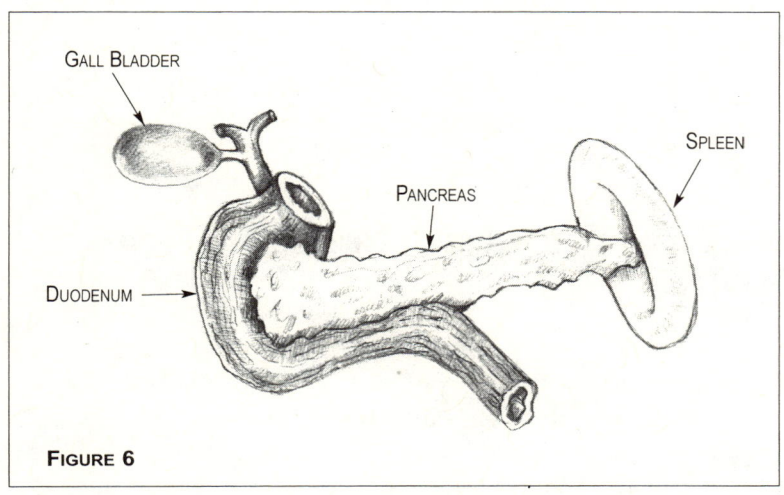

GALL BLADDER

SPLEEN

PANCREAS

DUODENUM

FIGURE 6

The duodenum and pancreas

The Liver

The liver is a large organ which is situated in the upper right quadrant of the abdomen. It extracts toxins from the bloodstream. It is the major biochemical powerhouse of the body. Most of the chemical reactions which involve the breakdown of small carbohydrates and fats and the conversion of carbohydrates to fats occur within the liver. The liver also secretes bile which when mixed with the foodstuffs which drain from the outlet of the stomach help in the process of digestion, particularly of fats.

The Small Intestine & Colon

The small intestine is a tube about twenty feet in length in which most of the absorption of food stuffs takes place. The natural ability of the small intestine to contract and relax, helps in the process of absorption and drives food on into the colon. By the time food leaves the small intestine to enter the colon, most of the digestive process has taken place and the colon merely extracts water from the effluent which enters it from the small intestine.

119

XX

Techniques Used in Surgically Treating Obesity

Surgical approaches to the problem of morbid obesity have existed for approximately fifty years and the number of procedures have increased at a very rapid rate over recent years. The field was slow to gain acceptance in the early years because obesity was considered by many to be not so much a disease as more a consequence of a lack of self-control. In recent years it has become apparent that morbid obesity can rarely be reversed by diet alone or a simple change in lifestyle. It is now equally apparent that modern methods of surgical treatment can not only result in massive weight reduction but also in an amelioration of the life threatening problems that are associated with the morbidly obese state. The indications for surgery are shown in Table 50.

Table 50

Indications for Surgery: NIH Criteria

- Failed Conservative Therapy
- 100 pounds over ideal weight
- BMI > 40 with no health problems
- BMI 35–40 with comorbidity

The first operation for obesity was carried out in 1954. A long length of the small intestine was taken out of circuit and bypassed. This resulted in the patient's weight falling from 385 lbs. at the time of surgery to stabilize at 140 lbs. This patient ultimately went on to further bypass surgery in 1971 and lost a further 50 lbs. The patient died in 1981 of a heart attack.

One patient had been reported in 1952 in whom a large amount of small intestine was removed and not bypassed and this resulted in considerable weight loss. In the early 1960s, several different procedures were tried, the difference being the length of intestine which was left in circuit. It became apparent that large amounts of weight could be lost by bypassing a major part of the small intestine.

Between 1962 and 1975 there were trials of several types of intestinal bypass.

Jejuno-ileal Bypass

These operations had various lengths of small intestine excluded which left intact only 40 to 100 centimeters. Bypassed small intestine was left in place and usually drained into the colon. The ultimate results, in terms of weight loss achieved with these procedures, were good but side effects were common, unpredictable, and often life-threatening, as a result of which these procedures were abandoned.

The various types of jejuno-ileal or small bowel bypass produced differing amounts of weight loss which was roughly related to the amount of intestine remaining in circuit. With retained lengths longer than one hundred centimeters, weight loss usually proved to be unsatisfactory. With lengths shorter than forty-five centimeters the incidence of protein malnutrition rose sharply. Some excellent results were obtained from this operation and long-term weight loss was sustained. However, the late complication of liver failure was especially alarming and led to some deaths. In addition, some patients developed electrolyte abnormalities in the blood which could lead to cardiac arrythmias and potential fatalities. Kidney stones, arthritis, gall bladder disease, hernia, persistent diarrhea and malnutrition with dehydration all occurred after these operations. Unfortunately there was no way of determining before surgery which patient was going to develop a malnourished state or any of the above complications. Jejuno-ileal bypass was abandoned, partly because of the high rate of complications. There was also a significant number of patients that did not maintain

121

their initial weight loss and late weight gain after five to ten years was common (Figure 7).

Jaw Wiring

Another early procedure was dental occlusion or jaw wiring. In this procedure the teeth are capped and the jaws wired in a fixed, slightly open position. It is impossible for the patient to take solid food and a milk-based liquid diet is prescribed. In some patients, approximately 60 percent of excess weight was lost over three years. The procedure was complicated by dental caries and problems with the temporomandibular joint, where the jaw articulates with the skull. A significant number of patients could not tolerate the procedure and insisted upon having the caps removed. All patients regained most of the weight lost after the wires were removed. In a number of patients the jaws were rewired and this was accompanied by further weight loss which again was regained after the wires had been removed.

In some of these studies a nylon thread was placed around the central abdomen and as waist measurements increased so did the tightness of the thread which produced discomfort for the patient, the thread cut into the tissues and created an additional stimulus to eat less.

The Intragastric Balloon

A device which was used some twenty years ago was the intragastric balloon. The rationale behind this was that the presence of a balloon in the stomach would create a feeling of early satiety. The balloon would restrict the amount of space available for food taken at meal times. The initial design based on this concept was the "Garren bubble." This bubble had a capacity of about 200 mls. and was clearly inadequate given the size of the stomach. The stomach has the capacity to accommodate about $1^1/2$ liters of fluid. It undergoes a process known as adaptive relaxation which enables us to eat or drink large amounts without feeling excessively full. This adaptive relaxation is a method of muscular relaxation which increases the volume of the stomach from about 50

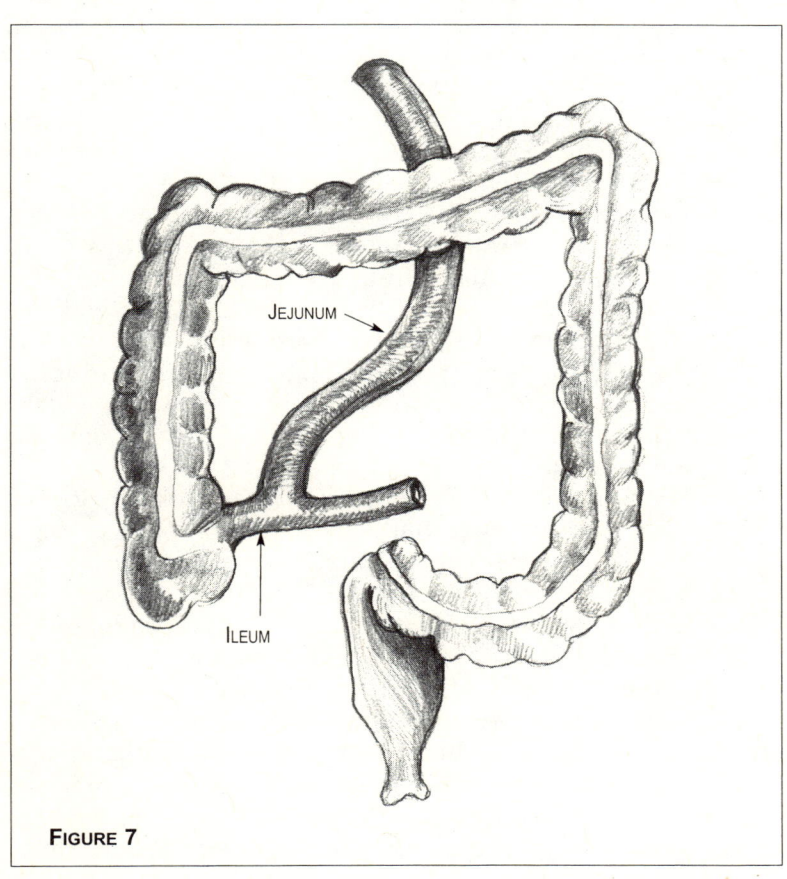

FIGURE 7

Jejuno-ileal bypass

ml, in its resting state, to 1 1/2 liters in its fully distended state. Beyond full distension, a feeling of discomfort arises and any further distension, after that point, will cause vomiting.

About twenty years ago, the author introduced the Taylor intragastric balloon. This was a silicone, free-floating balloon, which encompassed the above concept. The Taylor balloon, however, had a much larger volume than the Garren bubble, about 600 mls. This balloon when deflated was packed in the end of a tube or introducer. The tube was inserted into the stomach and through an inner tube the balloon was filled with fluid. A small amount of radio opaque material was introduced into the balloon so that it could be seen under x-ray. Fluid was introduced into the balloon and it expanded and came out of the tube which was used for introduction. When 600 ml of fluid was inserted, the inner tube used for inflation was removed from a valve in the wall of the balloon and the balloon was left free floating in the stomach. This balloon did create the feeling of early satiety and weight loss was recorded over a two- to three-month period. However, after this time, no further weight loss was recorded and in some patients weight gain occurred.

On reflection, even the Taylor balloon was probably too small. The concept of an intragastric balloon as a method of treating obesity is not all together inappropriate. In view of the stomach's ability to expand to a volume of about 1 1/2 liters, it would appear that the early research done in this field employed balloons which were of an inadequate volume to achieve the desired result. It is conceivable that if a balloon with a volume in excess of one liter were used, the results would improve. New materials are now available such as Melinex which can be extremely thin and is capable of marked expansion within the stomach. The material is inert and it is not likely to cause problems within the stomach. If an adequate amount of space is taken up in the stomach, then the ability to eat around the balloon would become increasingly difficult and therefore weight would be lost in the same way as it is lost with gastric restrictive procedures which are discussed below.

Gastroplasty

Gastric restrictive procedures are designed to limit the intake of food by creating a small gastric pouch. This is a method by which the stomach is partitioned using staples to create a small upper pouch which empties slowly, either into the lower normal stomach or into a loop of small intestine which is joined onto the pouch. Gastric restrictive procedures were introduced by Dr. Mason of Iowa in the early 1970s. When they evolved, it became apparent that the size of the small gastric pouch could only be something of the order of 20 to 30 milliliters. This resulted in gastric pouch distension after eating only a very small amount of food and the feeling of fullness stopped the patient from further eating. Should the patient continue to eat under these circumstances, vomiting occurred. When gastroplasty alone is performed, it does not bypass any part of the intestinal tract. This small pouch of stomach empties through a very small opening so that the rate of gastric emptying of food into the lower stomach or intestine is slow and therefore the feeling of satiety persists for some time. The physical restriction of eating caused by gastroplasty requires patients to ingest three to six small meals per day.

Patients are encouraged to eat solid food as by sipping high-calorie drinks or eating ice cream they can to some extent overcome the effects of the gastroplasty. People who drink high-calorie liquids in association with gastroplasty are prone to develop "dumping." One of the problems with early gastroplasty was that the gastric outlet tended to stretch with time and therefore allow more rapid gastric emptying than was optimal. To overcome this the gastric outlet was frequently banded by using synthetic materials such as Dacron, Marlex or silicone.

Vertical-Banded and Ring Gastroplasty

Gastroplasties interfere with the physiology of eating to a lesser extent than jejuno-ileal bypass procedures. Their evolution over recent years culminated in the development of two major types of open procedure; the vertical-banded gastroplasty and the silastic ring, vertical gastroplasty. In the vertical-banded gastroplasty, four layers of staples are placed parallel to the lesser curvature of the stomach and in the outlet of the gastroplasty a hole is punched through the stomach to create a new outlet (Figure 8). This outlet is reinforced by a band 5 to 5.5 centimeters in length

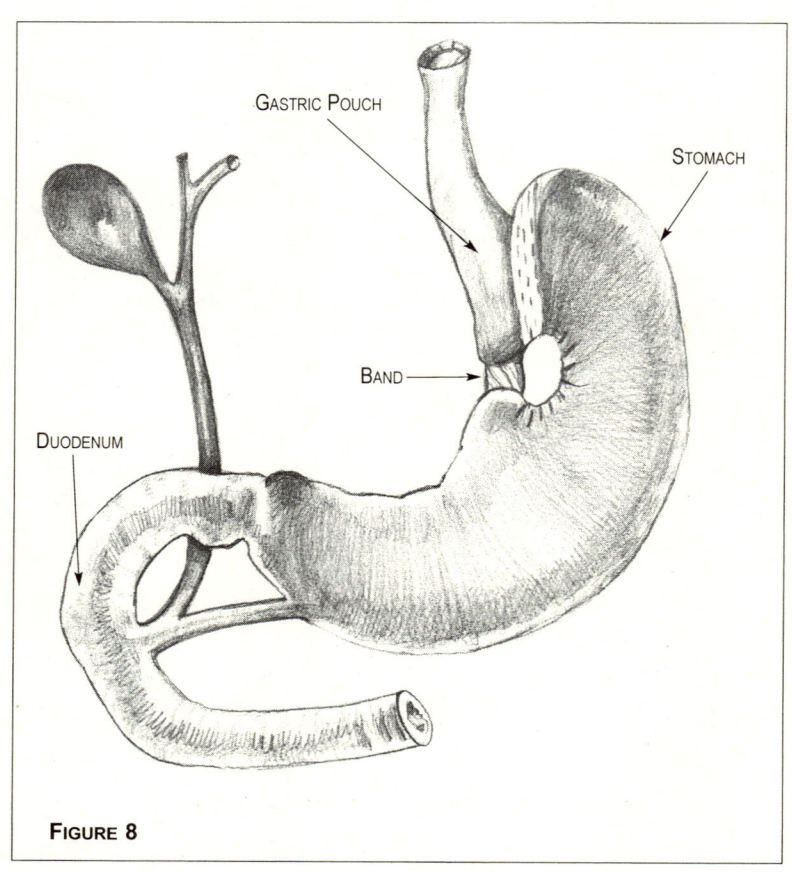

GASTRIC POUCH

STOMACH

BAND

DUODENUM

FIGURE 8

Vertical banded gastroplasty

126

which prevents the outlet from stretching. The total volume of the gastroplasty is of the order of 20 ml.

The silastic ring vertical gastroplasty is achieved by placing four layers of staples parallel to the lesser curvature of the stomach and placing a silastic ring around these at the gastric outlet, thus creating a new gastric outlet. This operation is performed by a specially designed notched staple gun. The results of vertical banded gastroplasty and silastic ring vertical gastroplasty are virtually the same and depend essentially upon the size of the gastric outlet and the volume of the gastric pouch.

The reason for the introduction of gastroplasty was that it was felt it would produce fewer acute complications than intestinal bypass. Vertical banded gastroplasty might have appeared safer and a less complicated procedure than gastroplasty with bypass or gastric bypass, but several studies comparing the two techniques showed very little difference in outcome. With gastric bypass, gastroplasty and jejuno-ileal bypass there is always a risk of leakage at the sites where the bowel is joined together and such leakage can be difficult to detect in the post-operative period. The patient's morbidly obese state makes examination of the abdomen difficult in the post-operative period and obesity also tends to delay the clinical manifestations of septic complications until these have reached an advanced stage, in which case they become irreversible and can go on to lead to the failure of vital organs such as the lung and kidney.

A problem commonly associated with obesity is gastro-esophageal reflex disease (GERD). This condition is virtually cured by the performance of gastroplasty as the small gastric pouch is incapable of generating enough acid to cause significant damage at the lower end of the esophagus. Furthermore it prevents bile from refluxing from the duodenum through the stomach into the esophagus. GERD is better prevented by gastric bypass than by vertical banded gastroplasty but the later procedure is also successful in ameliorating the symptoms of most patients who have obesity and GERD. The major advantage of vertical banded gastroplasty over gastric bypass is that it is easier to perform. Furthermore it is not associated with vitamin and iron deficiency or with the dumping syndrome. In the dumping syndrome the patient primarily experiences a sensation of light headedness which is due to rapid emptying of the stomach. All forms of gastroplasty result in an incidence of retention of solid food, sometimes leading to gastric outlet obstruction which may require endoscopy and the clearance of the obstructing debris.

Studies which compared gastric bypass with vertical banded gastroplasty seemed to show a greater weight loss with the former procedure. Weight loss after vertical-banded gastroplasty was on the whole something of the order of 60 percent of excess body weight at two years and 50 percent at three years. After a gastric by-pass patients lost between 65 percent of expected body weight at two years and 63 percent at three years. After this period of time there was a tendency for these groups of patients to begin to gain weight. This weight gain may be due either to stretching of the pouch with the resulting increased volume of gastric reservoir, widening of the gastric outlet, or alternatively, erosion of staples along the line of the gastroplasty.

Gastric Banding

In the late 1980s the concept of placing a band of non-expandable material around the upper stomach was introduced. Surgeons initially used a band of silicone tubing or polypropylene mesh to reinforce the outlet, creating approximately a 50–ml volume. This was tied around a "bougie" or tube placed in the stomach to control the size of the gastric outlet. The advantage of these procedures was their simplicity and the lack of any anastomosis which might ultimately breakdown and give rise to serious complications.

The Lap-band

Several groups of surgeons used non-adjustable gastric banding for a number of years and this led to a significant incidence of gastric outlet obstruction. An attempt to overcome the problem of outlet obstruction was made by introducing adjustable gastric banding. The principle of this procedure involved the use of a balloon, in relation to the gastric band, which could be adjusted so as to alter the size of the outlet of the gastric pouch. The adjustable gastric band was available in Europe for some years before it gained popularity. The reason for its popularity chiefly related to the simplicity of insertion and the reduction in complications associated with the procedure.

A further advantage was that the procedure could be performed laparoscopically, which led to shorter hospital stays and a more rapid post-operative period of recovery. Trials in the United States were initiated with the adjustable gastric band implanting a modified device known as the Lap-band. This was approved by the FDA as an obesity treatment in June, 2001 on the basis of a pre-market approval application that contained data from a trial of more than 290 morbidly obese Americans, plus international data collected in Australia, Europe and Mexico. This trial demonstrated that more than 70 percent of these patients who were followed for three years lost, and maintained, an average of more than 18 percent of their initial body weight. This weight loss represented some 40 percent of their excess body weight which, in many ways, was not too impressive (Figure 9).

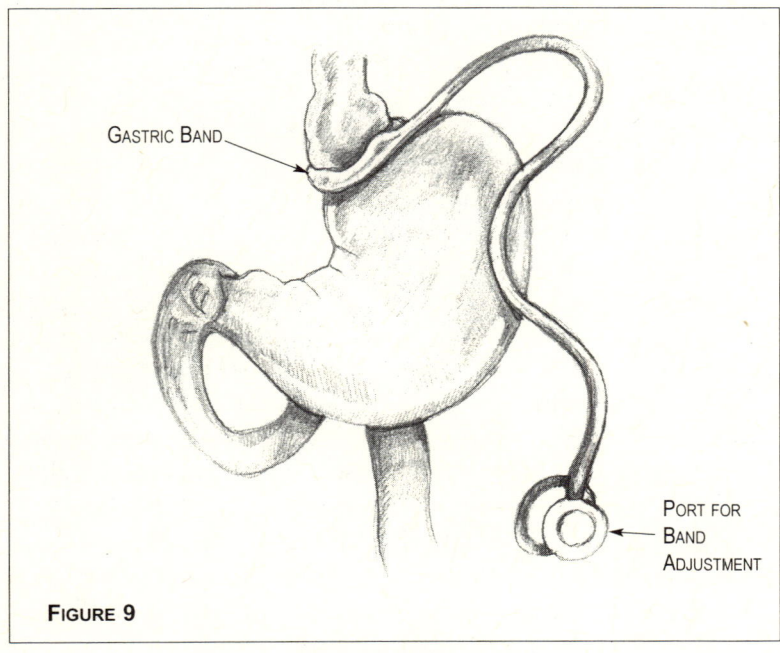

GASTRIC BAND

PORT FOR BAND ADJUSTMENT

FIGURE 9

The Lap-band

Variable results have been obtained with the band. The big advantage of the adjustable band has been the decreased hospital stays and shorter operative times. The band however is not without complications. Early in the placement experience with the band almost 20 percent of bands migrated or the pouch or esophagus dilated in the first year after placement. Techniques have now been modified to reduce this complication rate, but the overall rate of complications and the long-term outcome of the use of the lap band are not yet known. Some controversy therefore still exists over the use of the band (Table 51).

Table 51

Advantages of Restrictive Procedures

—Simpler to perform
—Easier to reverse
—Preserves normal GI tract route
—Better absorption of micronutrients
—Access to distal stomach

The basic techniques for successfully placing an adjustable gastric band rely upon: The creation of a suitably sized pouch close to the junction of the esophagus and the upper stomach; minimal trauma along the stomach while tunneling behind it; avoiding damage to the band while placing it around the stomach; and finally, creating a tension-free band which is uniformly placed around all of the upper stomach. Band slippage may be a problem and the best way to avoid this is for the surgeon to be very precise in the site at which he chooses to place the band around the stomach. The band should encircle an area of the stomach that is less than twenty milliliters in volume. Finally, the lower stomach is folded over the band to create a loose tunnel. This can be done by placing a few sutures in the stomach wall.

An additional advantage of the adjustable band is that it is relatively simple to reverse, although clearly reversal for patients who have undergone weight loss surgery usually results in a return to the pre-operative weight, despite the patient trying to convince the surgeon that this will not be the case.

Gastric Bypass—The Roux-en-Y Technique

When gastric bypass was first introduced, weight loss was variable and patients complained of bile vomiting and reflux disease due to bile washing back into the stomach. This led to the development of the Roux-en-Y Gastroplasty. Here the gastric pouch must be small, ten to thirty ccs; the outlet of the pouch should be about one centimeter in diameter. Bile should be diverted to a point lower down the intestinal tract and the loop of the small bowel draining the gastric pouch should be a minimum of sixty centimeters in length, before it is joined by the point at which the bile enters. Of these factors, probably the most important are the presence of a small gastric pouch and the diversion of bile in a fashion described as the Roux-en-Y technique, which had been described by the Swiss surgeon Roux in the early years of the twentieth century (Figure 10).

The Roux loop, as it is referred to, not only prevents bile from entering the stomach and thereby causing vomiting and pain but also for some reason not yet fully understood, causes a reduction in appetite and slows gastric emptying. Thus the combination of a small gastric pouch and a Roux-en-Y anastomosis has turned out to be the most efficacious way of achieving weight loss in the morbidly obese patient and this operation should be regarded as the "gold standard" against which other operations must be compared. Results, in terms of weight loss, are superior to those which can be achieved by the adjustable gastric band. In stark contrast to the band however, this is a major operative procedure which involves the creation of several anastomoses or areas where the bowel has to be divided and joined together. Wherever an anastomosis occurs there is a potential for leakage and leakage is potentially fatal.

Over the past decade the sophistication of procedures which can be performed laparoscopically has increased dramatically and it is now possible, safely to perform a Roux-en-Y gastric bypass with a low morbidity and mortality. However, the risk of this procedure in the morbidly obese patient should never be underestimated. Overall, a significant number of complications and deaths have been recorded and this is leading the American Society of Bariatric Surgeons to look more carefully, both at who performs

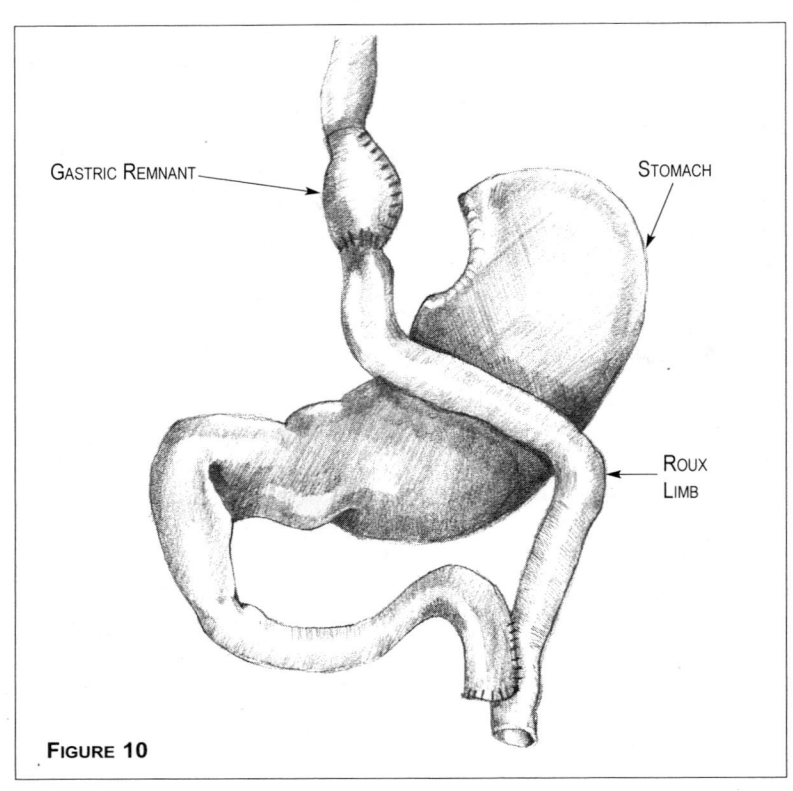

GASTRIC REMNANT

STOMACH

ROUX LIMB

FIGURE 10

The Roux-en-Y gastroplasty

these procedures and where they are carried out. Clearly there is something to be said for the development of a specialized "bariatric center" where surgeons devote themselves entirely to the performance of bariatric surgery: on the grounds that, "the more procedures one does, the better one becomes." This would appear to be a significant and powerful argument in favor of the creation of such centers and the development of a specialty of bariatric surgery. Whether or not this occurs will probably be determined in the next decade.

Indications for Roux-en-Y Gastric Bypass

The indications for gastric bypass are: 1) the patient should have a body mass index of greater than or equal to 40 or a body mass index in excess of 35 in a patient who has co-morbidity such as, for example, sleep apnea or diabetes; 2) the patient should be willing to undergo a period of long-term follow-up and compliance with medical treatment so as to avoid potential nutritional side effects; 3) the patient must be capable of understanding the nature of the procedure which is being performed and its potential consequences and should be well enough informed to give to meaningful informed consent; 4) there must be no history of alcohol or substance abuse; 5) the presence of any major psychiatric disorder, especially depression associated with suicidal ideations, is a contraindication. Other contraindications include serious medical conditions which increase the risk of surgery, lack of family support, and failure to understand the constraints placed upon a patient who has undergone such surgery.

Outcomes

The procedure of Roux-en-Y gastric bypass can vary considerably from surgeon to surgeon, for example, it may be done as an open operation or laparoscopically (Figure 11). The sizes of the gastric pouch vary. The length of the Roux loop also can differ and create varying results. The addition or absence of some form of gastric outlet ring or constraint device can also vary. The method of carrying out anastomosis of the bowel can vary between stapling and hand-sewn techniques and the length and nature of the intestinal loops and where they are placed in relation to the colon can also vary. Many versions of this procedure exist, probably the most reliable is that which creates a 20- to 30-ml stapled gastric pouch, a 1-centimeter gastro enterostomy, which is hand-sewn, and a 40 to 60 centimeter Roux loop. This is major surgery and when carried out in the morbidly obese the risks of anesthesia and surgery are considerably higher than for similar procedures carried out in those of who are of normal weight. There is a peri-operative mortality with this procedure which is of the order of 1 percent, in the best of hands. The most common cause of death is sepsis in relation to leakage at the site of joining up the bowel. Other causes of mortality are myocardial infarction and pulmonary embolism. Respiratory failure can also occur, particularly in the super obese.

Results

Excellent results in terms of weight control have been reported with this procedure. From a mean pre-operative weight of 300 lbs. the average weight after one year is of the order of 190 lbs. After one year the weight usually stabilizes below this level but few achieve the ideal range of weight, however the loss of 100 lbs or more is very significant to their lifestyle and to their associated medical problems.

Most of the patients undergoing this form of surgery are female and the mortality in males tends to be higher, also the results are not quite as good as in the female. Patients over the age of fifty-five have about a three-fold increased mortality rate associated with the surgery. Following laparoscopic gastric bypass the results in terms of weight loss are similar to those achieved with the open operation. It must be realized, however, that any procedure performed laparoscopically involves an additional dimension of difficulty when compared to the open route. The main reasons for mortality following the laparoscopic approach have, again, been sepsis due principally to leakage of the bowel at the anastomosis. By and large laparoscopic surgery is associated with a longer operative time, but with less blood loss and possibly a

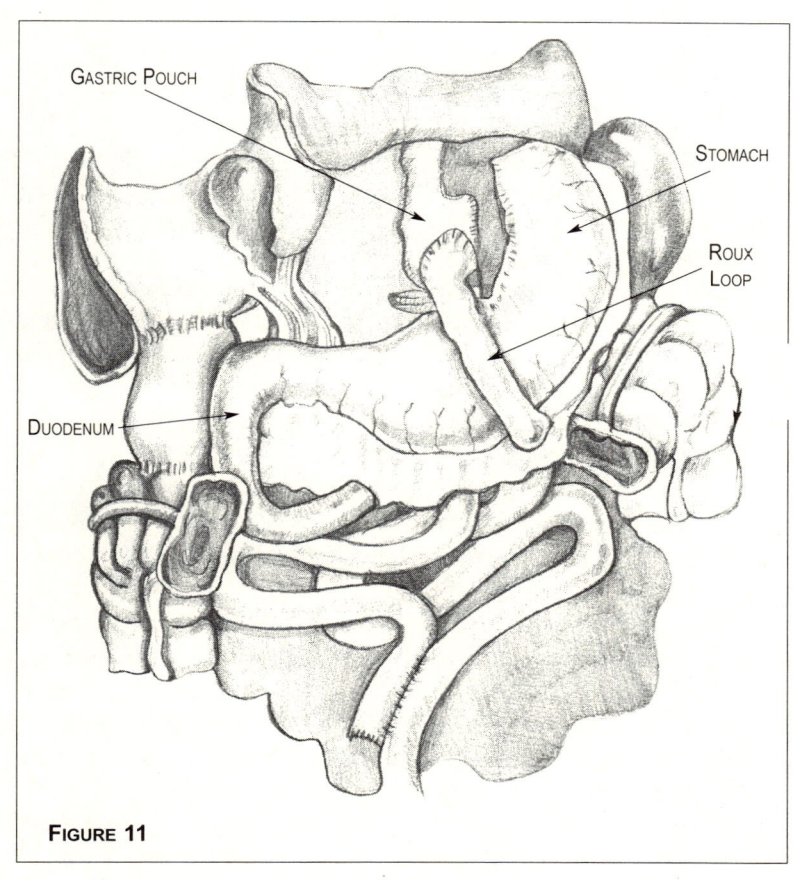

FIGURE 11

A typical construction of the Roux-en-Y gastroplasty

shorter hospital stay with a faster convalescence. The weight loss at one year is comparable between open and laparscopically performed procedures. One major advantage of laparoscopic approach is that there are fewer wound problems thereafter.

Long-term Advantages

Following surgery, full remission of Type-II diabetes, asthma, hypertension, infertility, fatty infiltration of the liver, gastroesophageal reflux and arthritis may be expected to occur. It is unlikely that in the future the mortality rate will be significantly lessened and it is of great importance that the patient who is undergoing this form of surgery must understand the risks associated with it. The risks of the conditions which are associated with the obesity however, in the long term, are much greater than those associated with the surgery and these risks are certainly minimized after the surgery. Therefore surgery not only greatly reduces overall morbidity, but the cost of medical treatment as well.

Biliopancreatic Diversion

As food passes from the normal stomach into the duodenum it comes into contact with bile and pancreatic juice. These fluids are essential for the digestive process. Pancreatic juice, in particular, contains the powerful enzymes, amylase, lipase and trypsin. These break down large molecules of carbohydrate, fat and protein respectively into much smaller molecules suitable for absorption. It is these enzymes which digest the pieces of steak you eat for dinner. In addition, bile is necessary for fat absorption and limiting its contact with food decreases fat absorption. When bile is diverted lower down the intestine, this leaves a much shorter length of intestine through which the food may be absorbed. If the bile is placed low down the intestine then malabsorption occurs. In other words all of the food products are not completely absorbed and some are lost from the intestinal tract. In this way, some of the calories which are ingested are not utilized. The principal underlying biliopancreatic diversion is to place the bile lower down the intestine so that a degree of malabsorption occurs. This procedure is combined with a gastroplasty and is used for the super obese patient. Two varieties of procedure, the Scopinaro Operation and the Duodenal Switch procedure employ these principles (Figure 12 & 13).

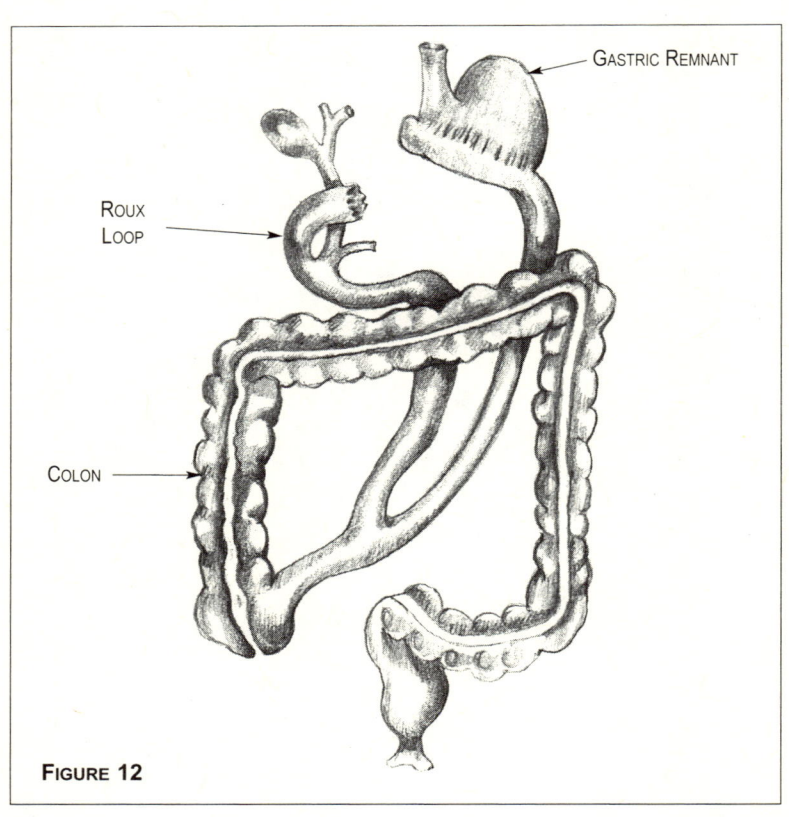

GASTRIC REMNANT

ROUX LOOP

COLON

FIGURE 12

The Scopinaro biliopancreatic bypass

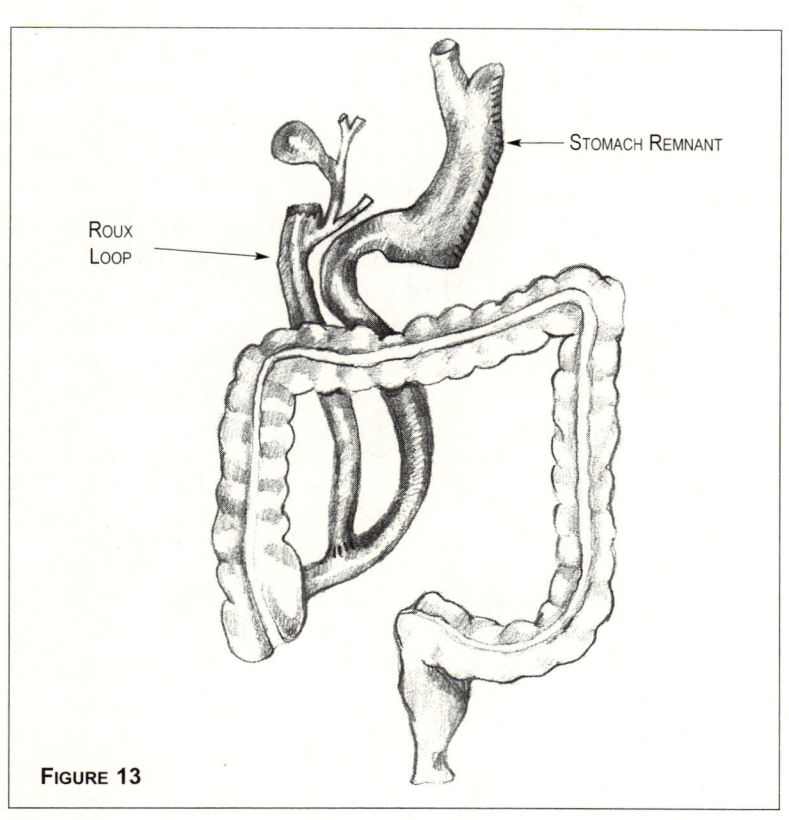

FIGURE 13

STOMACH REMNANT

ROUX
LOOP

The duodenal switch procedure

139

XXI
Gastric Pacing

Although surgery offers the best long-term results for the morbidly obese patient, it is major and carries considerable risk. As a result, more conservative methods have been investigated. It is now estimated that approximately 100,000 operations for morbid obesity will be performed annually, but the overall prevalence of the disease in the United States is something of the order of six million. Therefore, only a minority of the people eligible for surgery are currently undergoing this form of treatment. In view of the considerable risks associated with surgery, there has always been an interest in the development of potentially safer and simpler methods of weight control.

Gastric pacing consists of electrically stimulating the stomach and early results have been encouraging. The technique can be preformed laparoscopically and is much simpler than the technique involved in gastroplasty and Roux-en-Y anastamosis. The exact mechanism by which gastric pacing results in weight loss is not fully understood. It is well known that gastric distention acts to inhibit food intake and that rapid gastric emptying is closely related to overeating and obesity. It has been shown that obese patients have a more rapid rate of gastric emptying than non-obese subjects.

Gastric pacing involves the application of an electrical current to the stomach to retard the process of gastric emptying. The pacing is retrograde involving applying a stimulus in the opposite direction to the normal waves of activity that are associated with physiological emptying. It has been shown in animal studies that retrograde pacing can be associated with the loss of about ten percent of body weight. Early studies in humans have been encouraging, though there have been some technical problems with the

140

pacing device. However, no significant side effects have been reported.

Recent studies in man have shown a mean weight loss of 32 lbs. after fifteen months and 42 lbs. after thirty-six months. It has been shown that with battery exhaustion weight tends to increase but the batteries are replaceable. In Europe, a larger clinical trial has been carried out to assess the efficacy of gastric pacing. The device is usually placed laparoscopically in less than one hour. Some problems were encountered with lead dislodgement. The results were entirely unpredictable although some patients lost a considerable amount of weight, others lost none. Clearly, this device must still be regarded as being experimental. The devices themselves need improvement but the approach is novel, interesting and safe and further evaluation is therefore required.

XXII

Complications of Bariatric Surgery

The vast increase which has taken place in the prevalence of obesity is undoubtedly going to herald increased mortality in the untreated obese population. This is already becoming manifest in health-related problems such as diabetes, coronary artery disease and hypertension. It has been shown that the cost of treating patients for the co-morbidities of the morbidly obese state is greater than the cost associated with surgery for their obesity. However, surgery is complex and there are risks.

The morbidly obese patient presents special challenges to the surgeon and the anesthesiologist and the health care team. Venous access is more difficult. Intubation at anesthesia is complex and airway management can be a problem. Handling and mobilization of the patient involves many staff and is often difficult. Overall special and more intensive care is required for the obese patient undergoing abdominal surgery than for those of normal weight. As stated previously, the mortality associated with obesity surgery is of the order of one percent. There is a mortality associated with all operative procedures. The definition of a post-operative mortality is a death which occurs within thirty days of the operation. Clearly, within thirty days of the operation some patients are going to develop heart attacks and other life-threatening problems irrespective of their surgery but equally, problems from the surgery can accrue and these can be life threatening.

During the post-operative period, breathing is more difficult and ambulation is often slow. This leads to chest infection, collapse of the lung bases and to the formation of clots of blood in the lower limbs. The risk associated with thrombosis in the deep veins of the lower limbs is that of pulmonary embolism. Pulmonary embolism occurs when a thrombus or clot, usually in the lower limbs, becomes detached and floats through the circulation to block the main arterial output from the heart to the lungs. Fatal pulmonary embolus is more likely to occur in obese than in normal-weight patients despite the use of low dose of anti-coagulant drugs which may lower the incidence of this life threatening complication. In patients who have arteriosclerosis, surgery presents a major stressful incident which increases the risk of coronary artery thrombosis and death associated with this.

A major risk associated with weight reduction surgery is leakage from suture lines where the bowel has been joined together, either by direct suturing or by stapling. Surgeons routinely test suture lines at the time of operation but unfortunately, post-operative leaks occur in a minority of patients and can lead to the development of peritonitis and death. Leakage can occur from any point at which the intestine is either stapled or joined to another piece of gut. These leaks may be difficult to detect clinically in a timely fashion in view of the obese state of the patient's abdomen. At the first clinical suspicion the patient must be thoroughly investigated and if a leak is identified further surgery is mandatory. A later complication which can occur at sites where the intestine is joined is stricture formation. A stricture is a narrowing of the bowel which leads to partial or complete obstruction; in association with strictures, ulceration may occur and that may in turn, lead to gastrointestinal bleeding.

Another potential problem associated with major gastric bypass procedures is internal hernia. In this condition there is an abnormal protrusion of a loop of intestine through a defect inside the abdomen. Such an abnormal protrusion can lead to either intestinal obstruction or, in the worst case strangulation of the gut with peritonitis. Further surgery is mandatory to correct this.

Morbidly obese patients have an increased incidence of gallstone formation. This incidence is further increased post-operatively. Some surgeons routinely remove the gallbladder at the time of performing the obesity surgery, but this of course creates a further potential for post-operative problems so it is by no means universal practice. Rapid weight loss in itself increases the incidence of gallstone formation which can give rise to serious complications like jaundice and pancreatitis.

The commonest complication following open obesity surgery is wound infection, which may lead either to a breakdown of the wound or to the development of an incisional hernia. The presence of large amounts of fat on the abdominal wall predisposes the patient to the development wound infections and when these occur they may become complex, abcesses may form and the wound may require to be re-opened and packed. All of these complications delay recovery after the procedure. This separation of the abdominal muscle occurs either as a result of infection or breakdown of the wound. The wound may require to be re-sutured or at best a ventral hernia develops which will ultimately need to be repaired. Repair of these incisional hernias in the obese patient can in itself be a complex procedure often necessitating reconstruction of the wound with the application of sheets of mesh to reinforce the reconstructed wound. One of the major advantages of laparoscopic approach is that wound problems rarely occur. There are, after laparoscopic surgery, several small "port sites" which occasionally give rise to either infections or post operative bowel obstruction. But laparoscopic surgery adds another dimension of difficulty to the procedure. Pouch size and loop length are more difficult to assess and precise switching is more difficult to perform.

Following gastric surgery, the control of gastric emptying is impaired and dumping can occur. Dumping is a condition characterized by sweating, nausea, weakness, palpitations and lightheadedness. It is due to a combination of fluid loss and hypoglycemia.

The use of the gastric band is associated with a number of complications, perhaps the most serious of which is displacement of the band. Displacement of the band is associated with slippage or prolapse of the stomach through the band and this can give rise to obstruction and the necessity for further surgery. Nausea, vomiting and reflux disease are also associated with the use of this band. These problems can to some extent be corrected by altering the degree of inflation of the adjustable band, but sometimes further surgery or endoscopic stretching of the outlet of the gastric pouch may be required. An occasional complication of the band has been erosion through the wall of the stomach.

The older malabsorbtive procedures such as jejuno-ileal bypass were abandoned because of severe side effects. The major of these were fatty infiltration of the liver which could lead to cirrhosis and liver failure together with electrolyte problems. Electrolyte derangements can be life threatening, in particular a fall in serum

144

potassium can give rise to abnormalities of cardiac function sometimes resulting in sudden cardiac arrest. Only a small number of patients developed these life-threatening complications but it could not be predicted as to who was most vulnerable; and therefore the procedures ultimately were abandoned although some good results were obtained.

In the long term it is of great importance that patients adhere to dietary recommendations in particular taking vitamin and mineral substitutes. Without these, patients are prone to establish vitamin or mineral deficiencies such as Wernicke's encephalopathy, scurvy, vitamin B-12 deficiency and mineral deficiencies such as calcium, zinc and magnesium. It is important that menstruating females take an iron supplement to avoid the development of anemia.

XXIII

Long-term Morbidity and Mortality in Morbidly Obese Patients

After smoking, obesity is the second leading cause of preventable premature death in the United States. It is estimated that there are 400,000 deaths attributable to obesity in the United States each year. The epidemic of obesity is not confined to the United States and affects most Westernized countries. The related co-morbidities discussed earlier in this text lead to physical and psychological problems together with premature death. Bariatric surgery undoubtedly produces large amounts of weight loss in obese patients but until recently little has been known of the comparisons of long term morbidity in those who have and have not undergone obesity surgery. There has not been, until recently, a population based study demonstrating a significant impact for surgically induced weight loss on mortality and the potential for co-morbidity.

A recent study from Canada has addressed these problems, testing the hypothesis that weight reducing surgery reduces long-term mortality and morbidity in morbidly obese patients. This study from McGill University Health Center compared the morbidity and mortality of a cohort of morbidly obese patients treated with bariatric surgery to that of matched morbidly obese controls who had not been treated surgically. This is a large study containing a total of 1118 patients who underwent bariatric surgery for the treatment of morbid obesity between 1986 and 2002. A maximum of six controls were identified for each bariatric subject. The single-payer health care system in Canada enables health expenditures and clinical outcomes to be documented for all citizens. A total of 5,746 controls were included in this study.

The surgical procedure used for the morbidly obese patients was Roux-en-Y gastric bypass. Costs of health care were determined by searching the National Health Database over a five year

146

period. Patients treated surgically lost a mean of 67 percent of their initial excess weight. In comparison with controls, bariatric surgery patients have significantly lower incidence rates for the following clinical conditions: cancer, cardiovascular and circulatory problems, diabetes mellitus, endocrinological problems, genito-urinary problems, infectious diseases, musculo-skeletal problems, diseases of the nervous system, psychiatric and mental disease, respiratory problems, and dermatological disorders. There was a four-fold reduction in cancer, a five-fold reduction in cardiovascular and circulatory problems and a five-fold reduction in respiratory disorders in the surgically treated group. During the period of study the mortality in the surgically treated group was reduced by 90 percent in comparison to the control group. The mortality in the surgical group included perioperative deaths which had an incidence of .04 percent.

Another way to describe the mortality data is a relative risk reduction of mortality of 89 percent by surgery that produced a sustained 67 percent excess weight loss compared with no surgery controls. During the period of study the total in hospital days was significantly lower in the bariatric surgery patients when compared with controls. Also, bariatric surgery patients made fewer physician visits in the five year follow-up period including the planned yearly follow-up surgery group. Bariatric surgery patients had fifty percent fewer hospitalizations and significantly reduced hospitalization rates for cancers, cardio-vascular and circulatory conditions, including hypertension, infections and respiratory conditions. In contrast, the patients in the bariatric cohorts had significantly reduced rates for hospitalization for digestive conditions when compared with surgical patients. Typically, on average, the total direct health care costs for the control group was 45 percent higher compared with bariatric surgically treated patients. The finding of significantly reduced health care use rates and total direct health care cost is significant from a societal and health economic point of view because the health care services and cost associated with surgery were included in the total cost for the bariatric surgery group. Total benefit for the surgically treated patient would be greater than 45 percent if indirect costs were in addition examined.

This is an excellent study which has great strengths, particularly relating to the selection of the cohorts. Matching of the cases and controls with respect to age, gender and duration of disease reduces the possibility of confounding from these factors because both are potentially associated with morbidity indices studied and with increased risk for mortality.

Furthermore, the random selection of controls from an administrative data base reduces selection bias and bias by indication that would have been introduced if hospital based controls were used. This important study has produced emphatic evidence supporting the implementation of bariatric surgery in the management of the morbidly obese patient. It is a direct pointer to the health care industry indicating that with the implementation of bariatric surgery and the encouragement of the appropriate patient to undergo that surgery, it is beneficial not only in terms of morbidity and mortality but also health care economics.

XXIV
Obesity—What Should I Do?

This text provides an overview of the major aspects of obesity. Specific advice needs to be tailored to the individual but general broad categories have been outlined which can be separated from a therapeutic point of view. Therapy is not only instrumental to treat the obesity but absolute to the management of its complications. Treatment can be divided into calorie restriction, diet, exercise, behavioral therapy, drug therapy and surgery. All are disciplines and strategies needed to be adopted to cope, in the long term, with the lifestyle changes which are necessary to achieve the goal of weight loss. Compromise is essential in all aspects of life and compromise here begins with the trip to the supermarket. If it is not in the refrigerator you are less likely to be tempted by it. The bottom line in achieving weight loss is that the patient must take in fewer calories than calories which are expended. All diets depend on this fundamental principle.

Food must be rationed, there are no hard and fast rules about the way this should be done but rationing or restriction in some form is essential. The Atkins Diet, which in my own clinical experience has produced the most weight loss of all forms of diets provides an ingenious way of rationing in the least painful manner. Avoid carbohydrates and you can eat what you want. Given that the initial premise of avoiding carbohydrates can be adhered to, then caloric restriction is easier than with any carbohydrate containing diet. That is because large volumes of food comprising only protein and fat are difficult to eat without carbohydrates. Present yourself with a huge plate of sliced chicken breast, no sauces, and no additives and you will rapidly tire of eating it. It will be difficult to consume. Perhaps bacon and eggs are more tempting but without any carbohydrate additives again intake is likely to be limited. So it is bacon and eggs for breakfast, if you eat breakfast.

Most authors of diet books emphasize that it is important not to skip meals. Remember, the overall strategy is to reduce calorie intake. It is important not to exchange the omission breakfast for eating late at night, that is really bad news. Create a curfew at 8:00 P.M. and don't eat after that, except on special occasions or when there are extreme circumstances. Drink water at any time in large volumes. Avoid too much caffeine, which stimulates the appetite but drink as much calorie free liquid as possible. Tea and coffee are okay in moderation but use sweeteners such as Splenda.

Lunch and dinner are necessary. Go for grilled foods and throw away the frying pan. If you don't have one you can't use it and this will help. Look at the labels on meats in the supermarket and go for the high protein with low fat such as turkey or chicken breast and white meat. Pork is acceptable but cut off the fat. Fish is excellent, again grilled without batter or breadcrumbs. Green and white is the color scheme of choice so add to the white meat or fish, green vegetables such as broccoli, asparagus, green beans, lettuce and brussel sprouts. Add olive oil to moisten it.

For white vegetables, onions are great, if you like them, eat as many as you can, but potatoes are bad, French fries in particular. The glycemic index of potatoes is high so they are out. Bread is also out, just don't eat it. Triscuits, particularly the lowfat ones are acceptable and Ryvita is good. Add some butter to these and also some jelly or jam if you are hungry such as blueberry jam, which is excellent, raspberry or black currant but not grape jam. Grapes are just sugar. The other red or black fruits are nutritionally valuable.

Desserts are out, while you are trying to lose weight. Alcohol, in moderation, is acceptable. Red wine is the best form but alcohol should be restricted to two drinks a day. It has been shown a small amount is beneficial.

A combined multivitamin and mineral preparation should be taken daily. The large pharmacy chains probably produce the least expensive of these which give comprehensive nutritional coverage.

Exercise is a very important adjunct to dieting. Walk whenever it is feasible to do so, try to walk three miles per day. Cycling is an excellent form of exercise, burning up to 350–400 calories per hour. It is feasible to walk and cycle for relatively long periods without damaging joints. This form of exercise is also less boring and the scenery can frequently be changed. Joining a gymnasium is excellent and working out with weights is good, it stimulates a reaction on the part of the body to produce muscle rather than fat and this in turn improves overall fitness, exercise tolerance and mental as well as physical well being. In general make every effort to stay active, getting out into company and mixing with friends is good. Sitting on a couch in front of the television watching fast food advertisements is bad and is the root cause of so much of the present day obesity explosion.

Medication can be helpful for those who are struggling to achieve success with diet alone. In the authors own clinical experience the drug of choice is Topamax which is not yet specifically approved by the FDA for weight loss though it is approved and is widely used as an anticonvulsant. In the author's experience the drug is safe and results have been extremely encouraging.

For those who are 100 pounds or more overweight, surgery is an option. Although there are risks associated with surgery, the risk of continuing in the obese state are greater than the risk of surgery therefore they are worth taking. The author's feeling is that the threshold for embarking on surgery will reduce and I predict in the future that more surgery will be done for people with a body mass index of between 30 and 40 whereas today the threshold is at 40. More minimally invasive surgical approaches are on the way and will be used as these are most likely to be associated with a decreased overall morbidity and mortality.

There is a high possibility that in the future new drugs will become available which will be more effective in the management of the obese patient and along with minimally invasive surgery the overall treatment of obesity will become more proactive and aggressive.

Appendix 1

The Facilities Which Exist in a Comprehensive Bariatric Program

The comprehensive care of the obese and, more particularly, morbidly obese patient who is being considered for obesity surgery requires a multi-disciplinary approach. It is important that dedicated, compassionate and knowledgeable staff work with obese patients. The whole team should consist of a skilled and compassionate surgeon; an experienced anesthesiologist; dedicated and compassionate support staff; well trained nurses in the operating room, ICU and on the wards, a dietician; a psychologist, and excellent administrative staff. The head of the team is commonly a surgeon who carries out bariatric surgery (Table 52). An emphasis of the whole staffing infrastructure should be the appointment of compassionate and empathetic staff with an in depth knowledge of obesity and its problems and also of bariatric surgery and its complications. A multi-disciplinary approach includes the medical management of co-morbidities such as diabetes, dietary instruction, exercise training, specialized nursing care and psychological assistance is needed.

It is essential that staff members give the patient individual dietary guidance, that they are capable of carrying out medical triaging and detecting the co-morbidities which so frequently exist in this high risk group of patients. They must be present to support the patient in both initial office consultations and subsequent follow-up attendances. The team should attend hospital rounds and familiarize themselves with the patient during the post-operative period. They must act as educators for other hospital staff who may be involved in a more peripheral manner in the management of these cases.

Table 52

The Bariatric Team

Surgeon
Dietician
Psychologist
Internal Medicine Physician
Administrators
Plastic Surgeon

The Bariatric Surgical Team

An important member of the team is an exercise specialist who has the ability to teach and help with the individual needs of the patients, notwithstanding and considering their limitations. The person should be capable of motivating the obese patient and optimizing an exercise program for them. This exercise specialist must be responsible for modifying the exercise program as weight is lost, and carry out education of the patient in an ongoing manner, with an emphasis on guiding them to build lean body mass.

Psychological support consists of helping the patients to understand the risks, benefits and responsibilities associated with bariatric surgery as well as identifying high-risk patients and particularly those who have co-existing psychiatric problems such as depression, which may have an impact on their response to treatment. Psychological support staff should be in a position to evaluate the level of motivation inherent in the patient and inculcate the patient with the responsibilities which are theirs, in order to achieve a good result. They should also provide post-operative support, particularly in the early stages.

The dietician must have a knowledge of bariatric surgery, of its complications and of the problems that are likely to ensue. They must be trained in the management of problems such as the dumping syndrome and they must be sympathetic and knowledgeable in advising the patient how to accommodate for the restrictions in oral intake which occur as a result of a limited gastric pouch size. It is also important that they supervise the protein requirements, make sure that the patient's diabetes is responding to the treatment they have received and they must keep a very careful eye out for any vitamin or mineral deficiencies which occur, furthermore they must be expeditious in their management of these.

An additional member of the team who is very important is the administrator or insurance coordinator, who takes calls from inquiring individuals, advises them accordingly; who is well versed in the complexities of medical insurance and in the strategy which needs to be employed to obtain funding from insurance companies. They must be able to field patient calls and deal with these and any financial problems which are related to the treatment. They should also be in a position to schedule surgery and make sure that the fundamental facilities for surgery are available.

Patient Education

Patient education is of fundamental importance to the overall strategy in treating the morbidly obese patient in the long term. The purpose of education is to maximize patient success potential while decreasing stress which can arise as a result of fear and a lack of knowledge. It must be realized that surgery is a huge event in anyone's life, in particular in the life of the morbidly obese patient. The support must be positive. It must be emphasized to the patient that surgery offers the opportunity for them to start living a normal life again, but also they must appreciate that surgery is not an easy way out and that there are risks associated with it, although these risks are usually smaller than the risk of continuing to live in a morbidly obese state.

Practitioners realize that bariatric surgery is a fundamental tool, but it is the teaching of the use of this tool adequately and to the best advantage of the patient, which is the fundamental issue in treating obesity. It is the professional obligation of the multidisciplinary staff to support the patient through the difficulties that are experienced in association with achieving the goals of surgery. It must be emphasized that the treatment of obesity is a team effort and each team member should be dedicated to conveying their expertise to the bariatric patients. They should be available and supportive at all times. Having said that, there is considerable responsibility which rests in the hands of the patients themselves and the patients must be educated along these lines and must realize the nature of the obligations with which they themselves must comply.

Complexities and Risks of Bariatric Surgery

The team must give an in-depth explanation of the specifics of surgery and the consequences of the surgery as they will be perceived by the patient. The risks of surgery and its complications must be fully spelled out so that the patient is under no illusions. Bariatric surgery is complex. There are considerable risks. There is a risk of mortality, though this is small. Although the mortality must obviously be kept to a minimum, some mortality exists with all major surgery and for the obesity patient there are difficulties from the word "go." For example, obtaining access to veins in order, to put up "ivs," is difficult. For the anesthesiologist to intubate the patient for anesthesia also may be difficult. Obesity adds another dimension of difficulty to the surgeon in performing the operation. It is difficult for nurses to move the patient post-operatively; and also for physiotherapists to work on the patients in the post-operative period.

The expected benefits to the patient must be clearly spelled out so that a positive attitude is maintained, not only by the patient, but by the supportive staff. Furthermore, anticipated outcomes should be explained to the patient. For example after surgery, it is usual to achieve, weight loss of the order of about 100 pounds in the first six months. This will be a very positive piece of information upon which the patient can focus their attention and from which they can gain a lot of reassurance.

Expectations

The long-term management requirements of an obesity program must be fully explained to a patient. This is a problem which requires lifelong supervision. Even several years after the operation there are risks of nutritional disorders such as vitamin deficiencies which can be life-threatening, thus it is important to emphasize to the patient that they will require some form of medical supervision for the rest of their lives. The long-term consequences of the surgery must be explained. The constraints on eating invoked by the surgery must be spelled out, with their social implications. The problems of digestion, such as the dumping syndrome or diarrhea need to be explained. Cosmetic problems associated with large amounts of weight loss and the amount of redundant skin which hangs on the body as a result of this need explaining. The patient must be warned of the psychological problems which can be associated with a large amount of weight loss, particularly in the marital situation, where for example jealousies can be created and marital relationships can be put under stress as a result of the inherent improvement of the patient.

It is valuable for the patient to attend an informational seminar or to be given by the surgeon a document or video, which fully describes all of the implications of their treatment. The informational seminar should be conducted in a pleasant meeting space. All of the staff members involved should ideally be present, they must be a professional, well articulated, sympathetic, and educated staff who are available to explain any questions which the patient may have prior to undergoing this form of treatment. The informational seminar could be regarded as a pre-operative teaching class which heralds a lifelong commitment between the obesity team and the patient.

Informed Consent

The patient should be given some fundamental instruction in nutrition, some of the problems which can be associated with the nutritional disturbances that can occur as a result of obesity surgery, and they should be given exercise guidance and overall program information which combines a description of the surgery, its consequences, the subsequent nutritional constraints and the exercise guidance program. It should be explained to the patients that they will be required to make office visits and a data-based

157

follow-up will be constructed on each patient. The treatment of obesity may change in the future and therefore it should be a commitment on the part of the management team to remain fully informed of the rapidly evolving changes which are occurring in this field, so that the patients, at all times, should be given access to state-of-the-art medical treatment.

The patient will be asked before surgery to sign an informed consent form. Informed consent can be given by a person after receipt of the following information: the nature and purpose of the proposed procedure or treatment, the expected outcome and the likelihood of success, the risks, the alternatives, the effect of no treatment or no procedure, and the effect on the prognosis and the risk associated with no treatment. The purpose of the informed consent is to insure that the rights of the patient are fully observed and to protect the clinical staff from risk or liability. It is assumed that in all clinics a properly constructed system of treating the morbidly obese patient exists and that attempts will be made to provide state-of-the-art medical treatment.

We are living in a time of increasing litigation and the area of obesity surgery is one in which traditionally there have been a high number of lawsuits. The physician, from the point of view of his own protection and that of his colleagues in the clinic, must, in obtaining the informed consent, emphasize to the patient that there are risks including a mortality associated, with this surgery, as there is with any other operation, and that everything possible will be done to avoid life-threatening complications.

The life-threatening complications are chiefly those of thromboembolic disease, which means the development of clots of blood which can occur in the leg and on occasion become detached from the leg, float through the venous system and block the outlet of the heart. This condition, of pulmonary embolism, is one which presents a potential threat to all patients undergoing major surgery of all categories but to which the obese patient is particularly vulnerable. Each year in the USA 200,000 lives are lost as a result of venous thrombosis and pulmonary embolism. It is possible largely to prevent this by using low doses of anticoagulant drugs and this is explained later in the section on the complications of the operation.

158

Other life-threatening complications include coronary thrombosis with myocardial infarction, because morbidly obese patients are more prone to this problem as they tend to have arteriosclerosis. Respiratory difficulties can occur as a result of chest infection due to poor inflation of the lungs and septic complications to which the morbidly obese patient is particularly at risk.

The informed consent used for obesity surgery is usually one which has been specifically prepared for this procedure. Obtaining informed consent is another method of insuring and documenting pre-operatively patient's understanding of the risk and benefits of bariatric surgery as well as the lifestyle changes and responsibilities to which the patient must become committed.

The informed consent usually outlines the indications for the operation which are in most cases and fundamentally a body mass index in excess of forty. The alternatives to surgery are explained and the anticipated failure of conservative alternatives is outlined. The results anticipated from the surgery should also be included. The patients' obligations should be outlined.

Some surgeons also use a simple true/false questionnaire, which is given to patients pre-operatively to allow the surgeon the opportunity to validate the patient's clear understanding of the surgical procedure, the necessary lifestyle changes, the risk and benefits and the implications of them signing the informed consent. Samples of questions included in a true/false type of examination are:

1) After weight loss surgery I will need to take prescribed vitamins for life; T/F.
2) Patients never get depressed after weight loss surgery; T/F.
3) A complication following weight-loss surgery is a leak at the suturing site which may lead to a second operations; T/F.
4) After weight-loss surgery it is necessary to have lifelong follow-up; T/F.

ANSWERS: 1, T; 2, F; 3, T; 4,T.

Finally, patients should be made aware of multiple brochures which exist, describing the nature of their problem and its treatment. They can be referred to websites which give all of the above details. Booklets are available in major bookstores describing the nature of the surgery and what the implications are. Some teams issue their own newsletters, describing the excellent outcomes which can exist in patients who have undergone this surgery and this is regarded as a good psychological boost for other patients who are becoming involved in the same program. Videos are also available which often show before and after results of obesity surgery and emphasize dramatic changes in lifestyle which can accrue from an excellent result.

Appendix 2

The Surgical Procedure and Insurance and Payment Issues

The relationship between the health insurance companies and the patient needing bariatric surgery is complex and sometimes strained. It has been shown that health care costs for those with a BMI of over thirty are twenty-five percent more than for those of normal weight. Once the BMI is above thirty-five the increased cost is 44 percent. Life expectancy for the morbidly obese is reduced by ten to fifteen years and surgery both extends life and reduces health care costs considerably.

Of the major insurance companies, PPO's offer different rules on coverage which can vary even from patient to patient. Blue Cross / Blue Shield of Texas excluded coverage for bariatric surgery from January, 2005, this may also apply in Nebraska and in Ohio there is a cap of $10,000. In contrast in Virginia, coverage is mandated.

Medicare is often used as a guideline upon which insurance companies base their strategy. Gastric bypass is covered if "it is medically appropriate," provided that the surgery is performed to correct an illness. Obesity itself is now considered by Medicare to be an illness and surgery is covered for those with a BMI of over thirty-five if a related illness, such as for example, sleep apnea, is present. Morbid obesity has recently been given a diagnostic or ICD-9 code of 278.01. For Medicare a second related diagnostic code used to be essential for eligibility. Many insurance companies insist on various riders, such as a five year history of failed medical treatment, as documented by progress notes written by the patient's primary care physician.

Physicians' office staff negotiate with the insurance companies through a process which may be complex and time consuming.

Specific staff are often allocated this task. They determine the coverage language and the amount of benefits available. They should always document these negotiations accurately. They should determine the selection criteria, the deductible, the patient's eligibility, exclusion language, the nature of the pre-certification process and the number of days stay in hospital which are permissible.

Table 53

Health Care Payers

HMO—Health Maintenance Organization.
   Differ from one to another both in coverage of and proportion of coverage.
PPO—Preferred Provider Organization.
   Very variable in their attitude to obesity.
   More freedom of choice of doctor.
   More expensive.
Medicare
   Essentially the government-organized plan for retirees.
   Often the guideline for other strategies.
   Now recognizes obesity as a disease process with a diagnostic code.

Appendix 3
What the Patient Can Expect from the Bariatric Surgical Office

The fundamental requirement of all members of the surgical team, in the management of the obese patient, is to show compassion and an understanding of the nature of the underlying problems. The team, as a whole, must be aware of, and sensitive to, the obese patient's often lifelong struggle with obesity and the difficulty living in a "cruel" society can bring to them, when they continuously present themselves, in social and professional circumstances, as someone who is suffering from morbid obesity (Table 52). The pressures placed upon the morbidly obese patient as a result of their obese state are such that when they present to the bariatric practice they are a special group, not typical of most patients who attend a general surgical clinic with a problem such as gallstones. These patients have spent their lives struggling with their obesity problem and have suffered an enormous amount of hurt and humiliation purely as a result of their obese state. They may, in consequence, express this hurt, as anger, fear, anxiety and depression. The patient's self-esteem and confidence are usually low, even though they might put on a brave face. The patient that has been overweight from childhood has most likely endured years of humiliation, name-calling, an emphasis of failure, been regarded as asocial and has been blamed for the self-induction of their state. These are conceptions which must be dispelled and the patient must regard the bariatric team as being a sympathetic and a supportive source of consolation and solace for the state in which they have found themselves.

The medical staff who are managing the obese patient must realize that there is a wide spectrum of personality types within the severely obese category. Intelligence levels vary very widely, as do aptitude and application. Some of these people are extremely industrious high achievers. Others, as a direct result of their morbidly obese state, achieve much less, and find themselves somewhat beleaguered by all of the problems which surround such a diagnosis (Table 54).

Table 54

The Bariatric Surgical Office

Care & Compassion
Consultation
Investigations
Preoperative Education
Informed consent

Studies have shown that with the weight loss which occurs as a result of surgical treatment improves, the patient's self-esteem and self-confidence greatly increase. Frequently, marital satisfaction increases, but on occasions, jealousies can ensue and there may be strains placed upon a marriage as a result of the attention which the patient has received and the improvement in their overall condition and presentability to society. There are those spouses who may feel threatened by such a transformation of their partner's appearance which may create jealousies and insecurities which can even put the whole marriage under considerable strain.

The Consultation

The initial consultation is usually done on a one-to-one basis between the surgeon and the patient. A full and comprehensive history of all of the patient's lifelong medical problems must be documented. The patient must undergo a full physical examination and at the end of the interview be provided with an explanation of the nature of the treatment, its full implications and the lifestyle changes which may be needed for compliance and success with this form of treatment. At the end of this consultation it is appropriate the other members of the team should see the patient to explain their own particular area of responsibility. At the same time the patient may be undergoing those investigations which are mandatory in order to optimize the outcome of major surgery, the investigations include chest x-ray, EKG, metabolic profiles, other blood tests which may be pertinent and possibly CT scans and other more sophisticated investigations. Having gone through the initial interview and having met the members of the team, the patient should then be provided with the essentials of their pre-operative education.

Following this it will be explained to the patient that pre-admission orders will be written. Patients are required to take a particular bowel preparation to clear the intestines and to optimize the outcome of surgery.

The Hospital Admission

Patients should be told when to arrive at the hospital and that they should completely fast for at least six hours. Advice should be given in accordance with the taking of their medications immediately prior to surgery. Some of these medications may be taken; some will be omitted depending on the nature of the particular drug but a period of least six hours of total fasting is mandatory prior to induction of anesthesia. When the patient presents for surgery, their paperwork will be dealt with, their vital signs taken, the consent form obtained. Intravenous access, which can be difficult in the obese patient, is used as fluids will be given intravenously for the next few days and they will receive some form of sedation in the form of a pre-medication.

Following the pre-medication, the patient usually remembers nothing of the procedure until they wake up in the post-anesthetic care unit after the operation. There, they should receive adequate pain management. Drugs will be provided intravenously and attempts will be made for early mobilization at the appropriate time. After the post-anesthetic care unit the patient will usually be delivered to a hospital floor or ward area for their subsequent treatment. Should the patient have significant cardiopulmonary or metabolic problems it may be necessary to utilize an intensive care unit bed during the early post-operative period until they are stable.

Part of the pre-operative education that the patient receives should include instructions on post-operative dietary requirements. It is usual that they will be required to take fluids only for a period of six weeks. Perhaps toward the end of that time, a little solid material may be added. Thereafter they can move from soft foods onto a regular schedule of vegetables, meat and other protein sources. They must avoid overloading the stomach, particularly in the early post operative period where there is a risk of staple disruption as a consequence of overeating.

As part of their educational process the bariatric surgical patient needs to be taught about "pouch size." Commonly, the size of the gastric pouch is as little as thirty millileters, which is filled by eating a couple of mouthfuls of food. Furthermore, the pouch is emptied slowly and therefore the patient will never be able to eat a full-size three-course meal again, but will be subject to the constraints created by this treatment which physically restrict them from overeating. Instructions should be given about adequately chewing food and not swallowing large boluses of meat, which can give rise to obstruction of the gastric pouch outlet. In the presence of such a small gastric pouch, the importance of maintaining adequate hydration cannot be overemphasized and the patient must drink small amounts on a very regular basis. Ultimately, the more fluid the better. An emphasis should be placed on the need for early ambulation after surgery to prevent deep vein thrombosis and pulmonary embolism. It is most likely that the patient will wear compression stockings which reduce the incidence of deep vein thrombosis and also will be placed on a low-dose of an anticoagulant substance. Before leaving the hospital, surgical wounds will be checked; any discharge should be cultured. The need for vitamin and mineral replacement will be emphasized and patients should be given instructions as to how to obtain these necessary nutrients. They should then be instructed to present back at the doctor's office after their operative procedure.

Postoperative Care

Specific instructions should be given for the patient, in the early post-operative period, to avoid alcohol intake and anti-inflammatory medications such as non-steroidal anti-inflammatory drugs and aspirin, which can cause ulceration of the pouch. The post-operative exercise program should be outlined in great detail. Patients should avoid heavy lifting, but should be encouraged to participate in as much gentle exercise as possible and walking is an excellent form of exercise. They should then not only be followed up in the clinic but given ready access to the support group.

The Support Group

It is of fundamental importance to emphasize to the patient that obesity surgery in itself does not cure obesity. Along with this they must realize that they have an affliction which requires life-long maintenance therapy. The multi-disciplinary team has the responsibility to provide this therapy and the education which goes along with it. The role of the support group is to offer much of this education and to maximize the success of the surgery while at the same time decreasing fear and anxiety. The patient feels much more comfortable with their post-operative state when they can identify with those who have had similar experiences.

An important role of the support group is to emphasize to the patient that they are not alone. They are in fact one of millions who have this problem but they are one of a smaller number who have had the fortune and the strength of character to undergo treatment, which is necessary for them to achieve a long-term good healthy lifestyle as a result of overcoming their morbidly obese state. Having the opportunity to mix with others who have had similar afflictions markedly increases the positive attitude which they develop towards their management. The patient then realizes he/she is not alone, empathizes with contemporaries and thus benefits from a marked improvement in self-esteem. They should be made to realize that they have access to a supportive environment which has the expertise to deal with any problems which might accrue and in all likelihood they can fully cope with those problems.

These support groups not only help in the early post-operative period but, in the long term, patients often relate having received assistance in obtaining jobs, and in getting back into normal social and professional lifestyles. There is some resemblance between the functions of the support group and that of Alcoholics Anonymous. The patient ultimately feels great satisfaction from hearing of the many problems encountered by contemporaries who have fought complications, and overcome them. The support group therefore goes far in enabling the patient to fit back into society, improve their self-esteem, to nonchalantly enter a restaurant or a theatre, sit on an airplane without the embarrassment of not being able to fit in the chair, of breaking it, or of getting wedged in it. Furthermore, social groups also provide opportunities for dating and for good and long lasting marital relationships. Frequently, the members of the medical team have themselves been treated for these problems and therefore they are empathetic. Emboldened by this knowledge the patient also feels more confident about the nature of the treatment which they are undergoing (Table 55).

Table 55

The Support Group

- Surgery Itself Does Not Cure Obesity
- Lifelong Maintenance Therapy Is Necessary
- Patient Can Identify with Others
- Encourages Exercise and Lifestyle Changes

Exercise

During the initial and subsequent interviews with the patient the importance of exercise for the long-term success of bariatric procedures cannot be over-emphasized. Prior to surgery for morbid obesity, exercise is virtually impossible for the patient disabled with joint pains and severe breathlessness on exertion. However, during the post-operative phase when weight approaches the normal range or when a significant amount of weight has been lost, the patient finds an improvement in their joint pains and also they develop increasing exercise tolerance. At this stage it is important to stimulate their immune system and carry out as much exercise as is possible within their own limitations. With time, the quantity of exercise tends to increase. Many programs have an exercise coordinator and this is an important asset. The coordinator must have empathy and understanding of the problems associated with morbid obesity, but at the same time must encourage the individual to work up to his physical limitations. The motivation induced by a good exercise coordinator cannot be over-emphasized. They are beneficial from the point of view of improving the physical condition. Furthermore exercise stimulates endorphin production producing an overall feeling of well-being and adding a more comprehensive and positive attitude toward the therapy. Exercise programs have a high attrition rate and the coordinator should continuously try to stimulate the patient to persist with the exercise program.

During the early post-operative stages, when exercising is a problem, resistance training can be very helpful. This helps minimize muscle loss and provides a method of exercising without undue discomfort. Exercise increases metabolic rate and overall leads to a reduction in blood pressure, cholesterol, stress, anxiety and depression. It is sometimes beneficial for the patient to have a notebook in which they log the nature of the exercise carried out and its duration and use this as an added stimulus to continue complying with the program. The exercise log will be powerful reinforcement to the patient for the success of the program and a great stimulus to continuing to comply. Both aerobic and anaerobic exercises are beneficial, the first from the point of view of stimulating the cardiovascular and respiratory system; the second with regard to maintaining muscle mass and preventing muscle loss while maintaining the loss of fat from the body.

Glossary

Addiction: A state of being dependent upon some habit, e.g., alcoholism.

Adrenaline: A hormone secreted at nerve endings and by the adrenal gland—epinephrine.

AIDS: A viral infection due to human immunodeficiency virus which depletes the patient's immune system or their resistance to infection.

Amino-acid: An organic compound containing an amino and a carboxyl group. The basic components of protein molecules, some of which are essential to life.

Angina: Chest pain caused by inadequate circulation to the cardiac muscle through the coronary arteries.

Anorexia Nervosa: A condition of loss of appetite, decreased food intake and often profound weight loss, most commonly seen in adolescent females.

Anticoagulant: A drug which reduces the rate of clotting of the blood (e.g. Warfain, Heparin).

Antioxidants: Agents which block the effects of free radicals, vitamins A, C, E and Slenium.

Appendicitis: Inflammation of the appendix which may lead to peritonitis.

Bipolar Disorder: A psychiatric condition characterized by extreme mood swings from mania to depression.

Body Mass Index: An expression of the degree of obesity. Determined by weight in kilograms divided by the square of the height in meters. Quetlet's Index.

Calorie: A unit of heat, the amount of heat required to raise the temperature of one gram of water by one degree centigrade.

Cancer: An uncontrolled proliferation of cells leading to tumor and malignancy.

Carbohydrate: A sugar or starch with a characteristic chemical structure.

Cholesterol: A fat or sterol precursor of bile acids and steroid hormones.

Cognitive: Pertaining to the operation of the mind.

Colon Cancer: A malignant tumor occurring in the colon.

Coronary Artery Disease: Narrowing of the coronary arteries, which supply blood to the heart muscle, as a result of arteriosclerosis.

Corticosteroids: Hormones secreted by the adrenal gland which influence metabolism.

Cushing's Syndrome: A condition of central obesity, osteoporosis, diabetes and skin changes due to excessive secretion of glucocorticoids.

Diabetes Mellitus: Impaired carbohydrate and fat metabolism as a result of insufficient secretion of insulin or insulin resistance. Type I tends to be juvenile and insulin dependent. Type II is on the whole non-insulin dependent and related to obesity.

Diverticular Disease: A disorder predominantly affecting the colon where out pouching of pockets occur causing bleeding or inflammation.

Dumping Syndrome: A feeling of weakness, dizziness and light headedness produced by rapid early emptying of the stomach.

Embolus: Sudden blockage of an artery by a clot.

Endorphins: Neuropeptides formed in parts of the brain which influence cognition, feeling and activity.

Fat: Adipose tissue which serves as an energy store in man and animals.

Fatty Acids: Molecules of fat which are either saturated or unsaturated Fiber. An elongated thread-like plant structure, poorly digested.

Free Radical Oxidation Products: Breakdown products of metabolism as a result of oxidation.

Gallstones: Stones which form in gallbladder bile, usually consisting of cholesterol.

Glucagon: A polypeptide hormone secreted by the alpha cells of the pancreas.

Glucose: A basic simple sugar molecule, a refined carbohydrate.

Glycemic Index: An indicator of carbohydrate absorption through the intestine.

Glycogen: A characteristic chain of glucose molecules linked in a specific way.

Gout: A form of arthritis due to excess uric acid in the blood which forms crystals in and around the joints.

Growth Hormone: A neuropeptide secreted from the pituitary gland which increases growth rates in children and produces a condition known as acromegaly in adults.

Hemorrhoids: Varicosities lining the anal canal.

Hormone: A chemical substance produced by the body which has a special effect on a certain organ or groups of organs.

Hypothalamus: A part of the base of the brain which controls the autonomic nervous system and some endocrine activity.

Influenza: An acute viral infection involving the respiratory tract, tending to occur in epidemics.

Insulin: A protein hormone secreted by the pancreas in response to glucose renal.

Insulin Resistance: A desensitization of the body's response to insulin.

Ketosis: A condition characterized by an abnormally elevated concentration of Ketone bodies in the blood and tissues.

Lipid: A fat or fat-like substance.

Melanin: A dark pigment present in skin and hair.

Metabolism: Physical and chemical processes which occur in the body.

Mineral: A non-organic chemical usually found in the earth.

Myocardial Infarction: Death of heart muscle caused by thrombosis of the coronary arteries.

Nucleic Acid: A high-molecular weight nucleotide polymer in DNA and RNA.

Obesity: An increase in body weight beyond normal limits as a result of the accumulation of fat.

Omega: The final letter of the Greek alphabet.

Osteoarthritis: A degenerative joint disease affecting mainly the hips, knees and fingers of elderly persons.

Overweight: An excessive increase of adipose tissue.

Pneumonia: An infectious condition of the lungs producing inflammation and consolidation.

Polycystic Ovary Syndrome: Multiple cysts of the ovaries in obese females who exhibit hormonal abnormalities.

Prader-Willi Syndrome: A congenital syndrome characterized by mental retardation hypogonadism, insatiable appetite and obesity.

Protein: An organic compound containing nitrogen widely distributed in plants and animals.

Pulmonary Hypertension: High blood pressure in the left and right side of the heart.

Retinopathy: Arteriosclerosis of the retinal arteries at the back of the eye.

Satiety: A sensation of fullness.

Saturated Fats: Typically animal fats which carry the maximum amount of solute.

Schizophrenia: A major psychotic disorder characterized by delusions and hallucinations.

Set-point: A point at which in the natural course of events a patient's weight tends to stabilize.

Sleep Apnea: A repeated cessation of breathing from lack of stimulation of the respiratory centers in the brain.

Starch: A large carbohydrate molecule, a polysaccharide.

Stroke: A cerebrovascular accident resulting in the death of brain cells due either to hemorrhage or thrombosis.

Syndrome X: The metabolic syndrome comprising obesity, hypertension, high cholesterol and diabetes mellitus.

Tachycardia: A rapid heart rate.

Testosterone: The predominant male sex hormone produced in the testicles.

Thrombosis: Occlusion of a blood vessel by clot.

Thyroxine: A hormone secreted by the thyroid gland which influences the rate of metabolism.

Trans Fats: A type of fatty acid considered to be unhealthy.

Triglyceride: A compound consisting of three molecules of fatty acid esterified to glycerol.

Tuberculosis: A chronic infectious disease caused by the bacterium Mycobacterium tuberculosis.

Vitamin: A chemical compound in the diet, the adequate intake of which is essential for health and deficiencies in which produce a recognizable syndrome.

Bibliography

Agatston, A. *The South Beach Diet*. Rodale, 2003.

American Society of Bariatric Surgeons. Abstracts from Annual Meeting 2004.

Andrews, S, Balart, LA,Bethea, M, Steward, HL, *Sugar Busters*. Vermillion

Atkins, RC. *Age-defying Diet Revolution*. St. Martin's Press, 2000.

Atkins, RC. *Atkins for Life*. St. Martin's Press, 2003.

Barnard, N. *Foods That Cause You to Lose Weight*. Avon, 2002.

Christou, NV, Sampalis, JS, et al. "Surgery Decreases Long-term Mortality, Morbidity and Health Care Use in Morbidly Obese Patients." *Annual of Surgery, 240*, 416–424, 2004.

Diamond, H & Diamond, M. *Fit for Life*. Warner, 1985.

Holt, S. "Combat Syndrome XY&Z." www.wellnesspublishing.com, 2003.

Holt, S. Enhancing Low Carbohydrate Diets. www.wellnesspublishing.com, 2005.

Holt, S. Wright, JV, Taylor, TV. "Nutritional Factors for Syndrome X." www.wellnesspublishing.com, 2003.

Kirby, J. *Dieting for Dummies*. Wiley, 2004.

Martin, LF. *Obesity Surgery*. McGraw-Hill, 2004.

Mason, RJ. "*Gastric Electrical Stimulation*." *Arch Surg, 246*, 841–848, 2005.

"Obesity." A Report of the Royal College of Physicians, *Journal of the Royal College of Physicians of London, 17*, 1–58, 1983.

"Obesity." *Time* Magazine Special Issue, June 7, 2004.

Olshansky, SJ, Passero, DE, et al. "A Potential Decline in Life Expectancy in the United States in the 21st Century." *New England Journal of Medicine, 352*, 11, 1138–1145, 2005.

Ortolon, K. *Putting a Price on Fat*. Texas Medicine, 2004.

Preston, SH. "Deadweight? The Influence of Obesity on Longevity." *New England Journal of Medicine, 352*, 1135–1137, 2005.

Scheuneman, M. *The Calorie Carbohydrate and Cholesterol Directory*. Chartwell, 2004.

Taylor, TV, Watson, A, Williamson, RCN. *Upper Digestive Surgery*. Saunders, 2000.

"The Low Carb Frenzy." *Time* Magazine, May 3, 2004, 46–54.